Better Than Good Hair

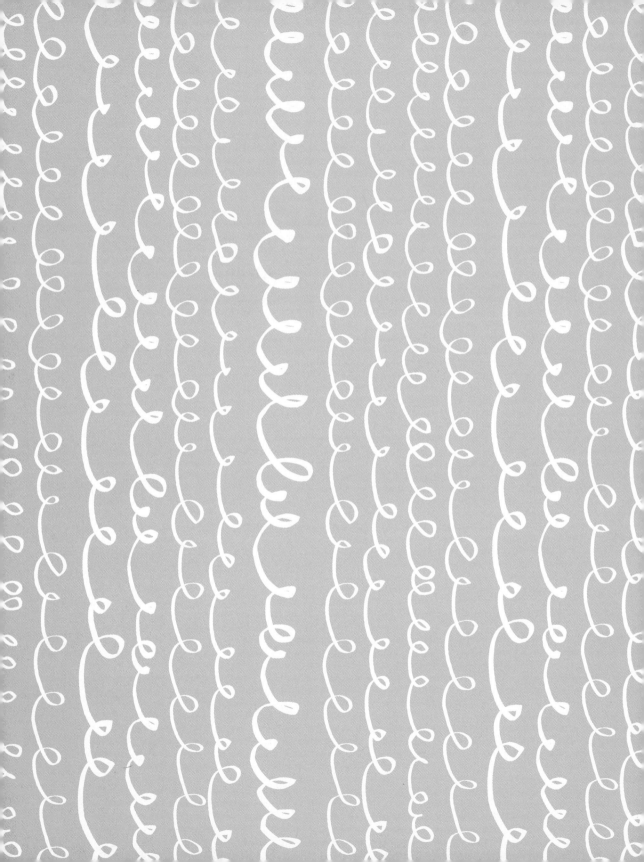

Better Than Good Hair

THE CURLY GIRL GUIDE
TO HEALTHY, GORGEOUS NATURAL HAIR!

Nikki Walton

MS, LPC, FOUNDER OF CURLYNIKKI.COM

with

Ernessa T. Carter

with
illustrations by Jessica Long

KICK THE BOX GRAPHICS

Amistad

An Imprint of HarperCollins*Publishers*

HarperCollins books may be purchased for educational, business, or sales promotional use. For information please write: Special Markets Department, HarperCollins Publishers, 10 East 53rd Street, New York, NY 10022.

FIRST EDITION

Designed by Suet Yee Chong

Library of Congress Cataloging-in-Publication Data has been applied for.

ISBN 978-0-06-212376-3

13 14 15 16 17   OV/RRD   10 9 8 7 6 5 4 3 2 1

To the curly homies everywhere, who shared my struggle and inspired me to be an advocate.

To my daughter, Gia, who keeps me motivated; my husband, Gene, who has provided constant support and guidance; and to my mother, father, grandmother, sister, and all of the friends and family who have supported me.

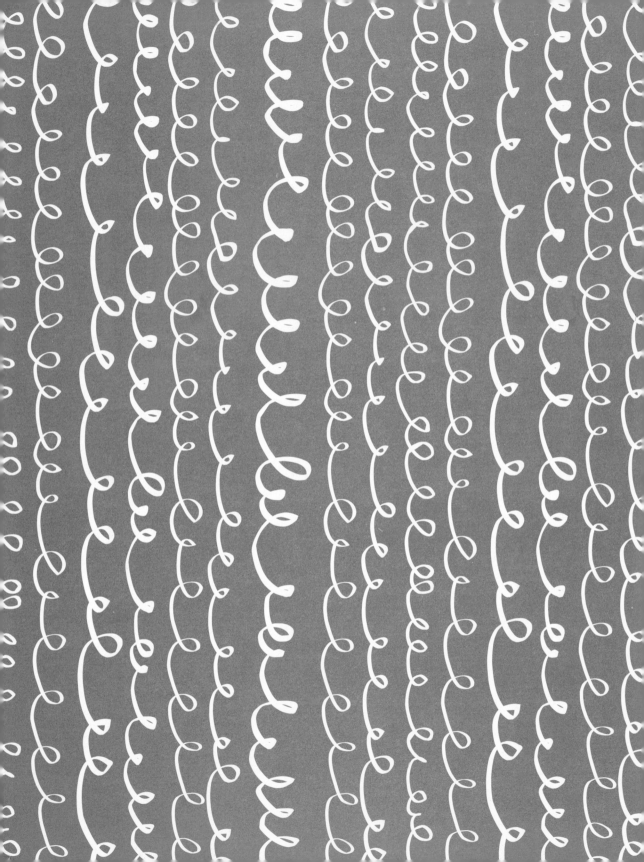

CONTENTS

FOREWORD

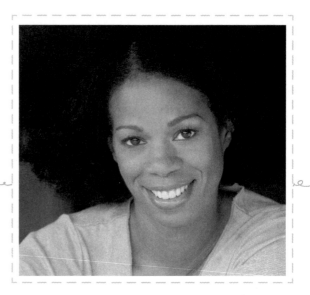

By Kim Wayans

The topic of hair is such a potent one. It's political, social, cultural, sexual, and, above all, *very* personal and emotional. How many of you at some point in your life have been guilty of canceling a hot date, calling in sick to work, or playing hooky from school because you just could not get your hair to act right? Maybe the weave needed to be tightened, or those unruly edges and roots were in some desperate need of the creamy crack. Whatever the case, you have to admit, hair drama is all too often front and center in the lives of women, especially black women.

We spend far too much time obsessing over our hair, and spend way too much money (sometimes the rent money!) trying to beat it into submission and make it do something it doesn't want to do. And who could blame us? With the mainstream media bombarding us with images of women with bouncin'-and-behavin' long, straight hair as the ideal beauty role models, it's no small wonder that so many sistas shy away from wearing their natural hair.

For those of us brave enough to consider breaking free from another culture's idea of what real beauty is—and finding our way back to our roots, so to speak—there's a great deal of fear around exactly what to do with natural hair. If you think about it, most of us didn't grow up learning how to take care of and manage our own hair. From a very early age, we practiced on our Barbie dolls (or her cheap ghetto knockoff, Shanequa) replete with straight, silky hair. In essence, we learned how to do nonblack hair. To make matters worse, we watched those television commercials where white women just jump in the shower, wash their hair without a hitch, then shake and go. If we tried that, we'd wind up with a matted bird's nest that you couldn't get a comb through for a week!

Looking back on my own hair journey, I was fortunate that I never had a perm. Which isn't to say I didn't want one. Like almost every other little black girl I knew, I was desperate to push the hair out of my eyes and toss it over my shoulder like Marcia Brady. But my progressive mother was not having it. She was adamant about her girls maintaining their natural hair while living under her roof. No matter how much my sisters and I reasoned, argued, or got down on our ashy knees and begged, she held her ground. We could hot-comb our hair if we must, but absolutely no chemicals were allowed in her house.

So the hot comb became my best friend. And it served me pretty well until it was time to go away to college at a predominately white university in Middletown, Connecticut, miles away from my hometown of New York City. I remember being stressed out in the weeks before leaving, worrying about how I would maintain my press and curl while I was away.

I thought I'd found a genius solution—buying an electric hot plate—until I almost burned down the dorm one night when my ten-dollar fleece blanket got too close to the apparatus and went up in flames. Luckily, I was able to snuff it out before it got out of hand. Rather than try to explain to all those clueless white girls in my dorm what a hot comb was, and why I was using it (especially since they had assumed that my hair was just naturally straight, and I'd allowed that fraud to perpetuate), I said I'd burned some popcorn instead!

From then on, whenever they would smell burnt hair and smoke wafting from under my door, I could hear them whisper to one another, "Oh, Kim's burning popcorn again. How hard is it to cook popcorn anyway?" Well, I'm here to tell you, Kim burned some popcorn once a week for four years. I'm sure to this day they're all wondering what the hell was up with the black girl and her popcorn.

After graduating and moving out to sunny California, I became more health conscious, so I joined a gym and started working out. I quickly discovered that I couldn't break a sweat without hearing the faint sound of African drums in my head as my kitchen started napping up. Well, sista-girl couldn't have her press and curl going back on her, so I did what most other women in my predicament would do—I gave up my gym membership. Hair that lay straight was simply more important to me than a strong cardiovascular system.

Eventually, though, I got tired of hanging out at pool parties, pretending that I enjoyed baking to a crisp in the sun without ever taking a dip in the pool. And I also got tired of running like a madwoman for the nearest shelter whenever I felt a drop of rain fall from the sky. A change was due. So

I gave up my press and curl and made the leap to individual braids with extensions.

I must admit I *loved* my braids. It was kind of like having long, straight hair, but I could exercise and even take a swim! And the tons of compliments I received from folks were quite addictive. People would always comment on how beautiful and exotic my braids were. I went from being a slave to my hot comb to being a slave to my extensions. They were quite costly and time-consuming, too. Every two months, I'd sit for eight hours to get them taken out; then come back the next day and sit for upward of fourteen hours to get them put back in. I could've bought a vacation home in Antigua with all those fat checks I was writing to the stylists to keep up my do.

The longer I wore braids, though, the more I discovered some of the pitfalls of wearing them. The most embarrassing was that an extension would often loosen and fall out when you least expected it. Like the one that fell out when I was standing in line at the buffet at my best friend's wedding. It plopped down right on top of the curried chicken, which wouldn't have been too face-breaking if the fine guy standing behind me hadn't lifted it up and handed it to me as I was trying to make a clean getaway. I have more stories like that than I care to remember. It got to the point where my extensions became like Hansel and Gretel's bread crumb trail. If you needed to find Kim, just follow the fallen extensions.

But even worse was when I started noticing that my edges were breaking off and my hairline was slowly creeping backward, thanks to too much stress being placed on the hair follicles from the weight of the extensions. Faced with the choice of either looking like Egghead McGee with a hairline that started back behind my ears or giving up the braids, I decided that the braids had to go. I needed a different style and quick. But what? I knew I didn't want to get a weave, and that was mostly because I had hugged one too many weave-wearing mamas whose head smelled like something crawled up under that weave cap and died. I needed access to my scalp, so I could keep it clean and smelling lovely. Moreover, I didn't want to become one of those scary women who would put a brotha in a choke hold if he attempted to touch her hair. (Weave wearers can be extremely sensitive to human touch.)

With much trepidation, I decided I would take out the extensions and go completely natural. This was not an easy decision to make. To be quite honest, I was scared. I had become so attached to my braids. What was I going to look like without them? Would I still be cute? Would people still compliment me? Would men still be attracted to me? It's incredible to think how insecure I was initially about wearing my own hair.

Making that transition caused me to do some real soul-searching. It forced me to ask myself some tough questions about my notions of beauty: how they were formulated, the value we place on hair, and what it is we believe straight, long hair buys us.

In many ways, going completely natural was a spiritual journey that enabled me to remove a mask and become my more authentic self. By reclaiming my own natural beauty and relinquishing the need to be a pale imitation of somebody else's, I had liberated and empowered myself in a very deep way.

The problem that still presented itself to me, though, was how to care for my own hair. My first couple of years as a natural were a hit-and-miss, trial-and-error (mostly error) period of experimentation and frustration because I was basically operating in the dark. I was constantly battling knots, hair matting, dryness, and so on. I swear, I lost enough handfuls of hair to make my own wig!

Fortunately, one day while moaning about my hair woes to my friend Robin, a fellow natural, she introduced me to what turned out to be a godsend for me (and countless other naturals)—a website called CurlyNikki.com. From that website I learned almost everything I know about how to care for, nourish, and style my natural hair. What a tremendous resource it is. It's not an exaggeration when I say that finding CurlyNikki has been one of the best things that's ever happened to me.

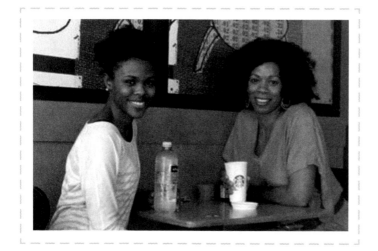

Armed with all the knowledge and instruction I culled from CurlyNikki, along with the fabulous product suggestions and hair tool recommendations, working with my natural hair became a joy and an adventure in creativity. So from the bottom of my heart, thank you, Nikki! Now, in retrospect, I laugh at all the hairballs I yanked out using those skinny little combs on my thick, coarse tresses. What was I thinking? It was like trying to rake a lawn with a fork. Black hair is different, and it demands different treatment to survive and thrive. Which brings me to the topic of *Better Than Good Hair.*

Needless to say, I was over the moon when Nikki told me she was putting together what is sure to be the bible on natural hair care. What exciting news for all of us naturals and wannabe naturals. A hair guide that will demystify the process of being natural with ease and answer just about any question that you may have about natural hair care. I wish I had a guide like this when I first went natural. This book is not only sorely needed but will no doubt help usher in the revolution of women coming home to wear their natural hair. Not just wearing it, but wearing it with pride. Sporting the beautiful, luxurious, interesting, thick, springy, curly, coily, kinky hair they've been blessed with. Come gift-giving season, I know what all my girlfriends and sisters are getting: *Better Than Good Hair*!

Our natural hair is versatile and alive with so much personality. It demands and commands attention, and it talks to you, if you listen. Open up those ears and hear what your hair is saying. Let *Better Than Good Hair* help you to embrace and unmask the natural woman who dwells within. Then bask in all the beauty, confidence, grace, and power it calls forth. Talk about compliments—you'll get more now than ever before! For there is nothing more special, alluring, foxy, and powerful than a natural sista. When you believe it, so will the world!

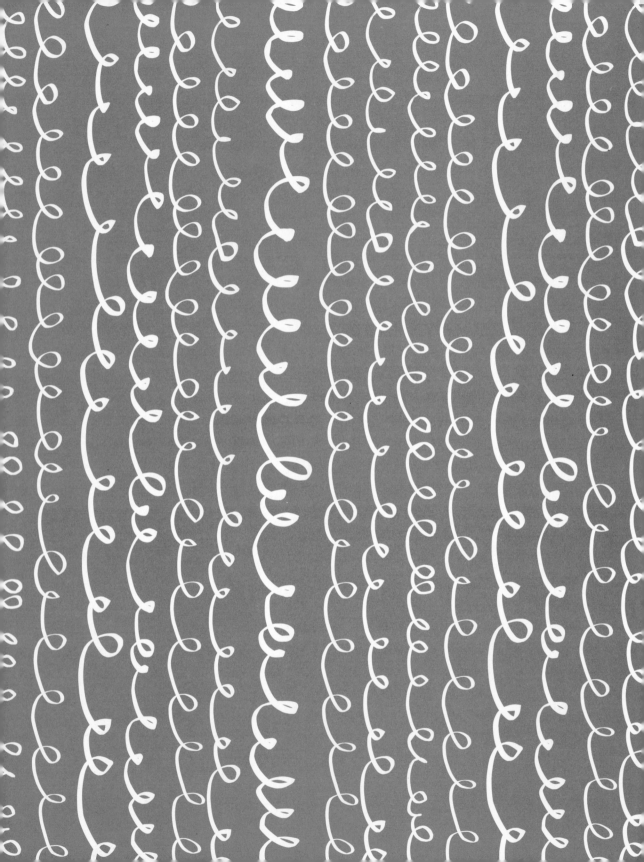

PROLOGUE

Dear Curlfriends,

I often get stopped on the street by other black women. They tell me that they love my hair and want to know who "does" it. It always gives me great pleasure to tell them that I do it myself. And it gives me even more pleasure to refer them to CurlyNikki.com to find out how they, too, can achieve fabulous, healthy, natural hair on their own.

But of course I didn't come out of the womb with the magical ability to do my own hair, nor did I have a fairy hair godmother. I grew up in St. Louis, Missouri, and though I had amazing parents, I suffered through an awkward adolescence plagued with self-esteem issues tied to my not-so-hot hot-combed hair. Before I turned ten, my mother and grandmother took wonderful care of my hair by simply washing and conditioning it and keeping it in braids. It grew to waist length. But I wanted bone straight hair, and my parents had banned relaxers. So between the ages of ten and sixteen, I went to a salon every two weeks to have my long hair blown out and combed straight. However, my hair never looked the way I wanted it to. It would revert almost immediately and end up in a frizzy, greasy, poofy mess.

Finally, late in my junior year of high school, my younger sister and I began going to a different salon. This place had young stylists and brand-new-to-us technology called *flat irons*—no grease required. When my new beautician turned me to face the mirror, I felt like my hair had been transformed. Awkward old me had been replaced with a much better version of myself. My hair was silky and flowing in the wind, and nobody could tell me nothing. I went back to school with a new attitude, feeling pretty for the first time in my life.

I soon became addicted to getting my hair flat-ironed every two weeks. My beautician washed my hair with a very stringent, moisture-stripping shampoo every session and didn't use a leave-in conditioner to give it that silky look. As a consequence, much to my confused dismay, my once healthy bra-strap-length hair began to disappear right before my eyes. As it turned out, my old system of sporadic press and curls with lots of lubrication was much better for my hair health than regular flat-iron sessions on product-free hair.

By the time I left for college at Truman State University (location: middle-of-nowhere, USA), my hair had broken off to a shoulder-length bob. But as long as it was bone straight, I didn't care. I loved my silky hair, and I could not quit the flat iron. I might have kept going on like that until it was Halle Berry–short, except for two things.

First, like many black girls raised in the salon, I had never even washed my own hair. I discovered that I had no idea how to moisturize it or even how to deal with it between sporadic visits back home to St. Louis, over three hours away.

The other thing that happened is that I met a young man named Eugene during freshman orientation. It was love at first sight. Gene was smart, handsome, and sensitive. Most of all, he loved me despite the fact that my hair was turning into an absolute wreck.

But as it turned out, it was more than my hair that was turning into a wreck. Two years into our relationship, Gene sat me down and told me that my mood seemed to be directly correlated to the current condition of my hair, and he thought that was unhealthy. He suggested that I start doing my own hair and wearing it in its natural texture.

Here I was, a psych major receiving a hair intervention from my boyfriend. And the worst thing was that I knew he was right. It wasn't healthy to obsess over my hair the way I did, to feel terrible when my hair didn't look good. But in the words of R&B group TLC, I felt "unpretty" when my hair wasn't perfectly straight, and since it didn't grow out of my scalp that way, I just couldn't take his advice in full.

I met him halfway by purchasing my own Solia flat iron. But then, what was supposed to be me "taking back my hair" became an even bigger obsession. I found myself hitting the flat iron once a week, sometimes more. Finally, with Gene's continued encouragement, I started using the flat iron less and experimenting with natural styles more. By the end of my senior year, I had begun two-strand-twisting my hair, rocking twist-outs, and even wearing my hair in puffs. At first I felt very self-conscious about wearing my curls out in public. But as time went on, I actually began to prefer my hair in its natural state. I didn't have to worry about Missouri's notorious humidity, and natural styles were easy to do. Plus, my curly hair made me feel special, like I stood out in a crowd.

In 2005, Gene and I moved to North Carolina to attend graduate school at UNC Chapel Hill (Go Heels!) and Duke. That's when I discovered NaturallyCurly.com, and my hair obsession switched from flat-ironing to learning how to achieve healthy, natural hair on my own. By late 2006, I had stopped flat-ironing regularly, and with the help of the women on Naturally Curly.com's hair forums, I nursed my damaged hair back to health.

Gene loved my natural hair. He proposed after we moved to North Carolina and actually requested that I wear my hair natural on our wedding day. I almost cried when he asked me that. He had been nothing but supportive, and truth be told, *he* is the reason I found the confidence to go natural. He made me look inside myself and see that the cause of my psychological distress was my irrational belief about how my hair *should* be. My hard-found self-awareness coupled with the education I'd received from other women inspired me to start CurlyNikki .com in 2008.

As of this writing, CurlyNikki.com is the most popular natural hair care blog in the world. We're presenting this book to you as a compendium of the knowledge we've gained these last few years.

Now that I've told you my hair story, I'll tell you what this book is not.

This book is not a political manifesto intent on shaming you into giving up your relaxer. We respect your hair decisions, and we support you in whatever path you choose to take with your own hair. If you want to keep your hair straight but are curious about wearing your hair natural, we're here for you. If you haven't decided whether to give up your relaxer, we're here for you. We don't even have one of those harsh relaxer vs. natural hair sections in this book. We only want to provide you with the information that you need to take the next step in your own hair journey, and we do not want to bully or shame you in any way.

We're also not antihairdresser. Though I love the freedom of doing my own hair for work, play, and formal events alike, I understand that many of you enjoy going to the salon. Feel free to share our tips and hairstyle guides with your beautician so that you and your stylist may continue on your natural hair journey together.

One more thing this book isn't: a memoir or a you-must-do-exactly-like-Nikki guide. The natural hair community is just that—a *community* of women; our coworkers, mothers, sisters, and friends who are embracing their natural hair and sharing their frustrations and triumphs. One of the things I've enjoyed most as a natural hair blogger is fostering that sense of community and providing a platform for folks to share. I've had the pleasure of meeting tons of beautiful, successful women, and for this book we've chosen to include a diverse group of real-life natural community members as our models, stylistas, and advice givers.

You see, most of all, we want this book to be a friend to you. Inside you'll find product guidance, lifestyle advice, hairstyle tips, and frank discussion—just as you would in any hair salon across America. We want you to know that you are not alone in your hair journey. We're here for you, and we can't wait to compliment you on how good your hair looks.

Later Gators,

Nikki Walton

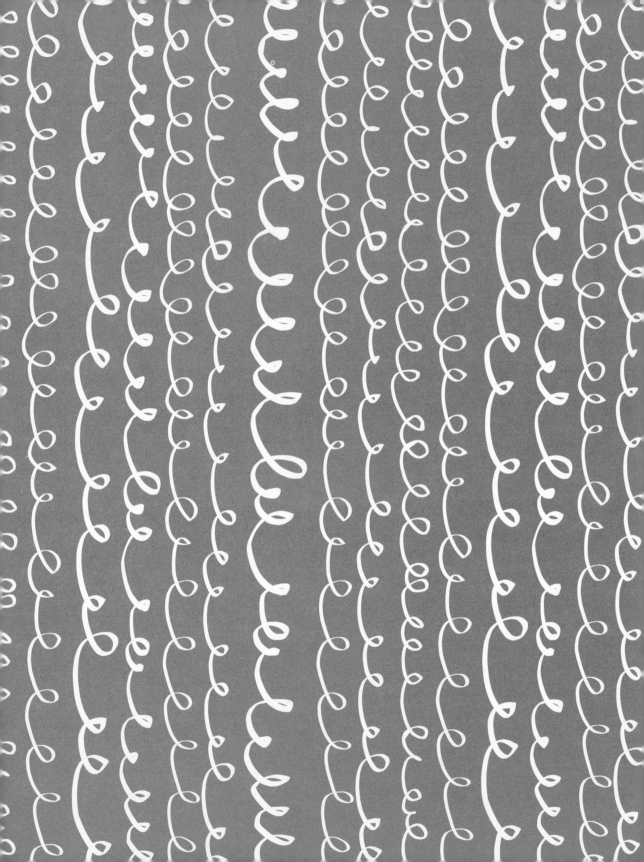

CHAPTER ONE

The Big Chop

Mama, Friends, and Significant Others (How to Transition Without Losing Your Mind)

For those of us with relaxed hair, the hardest step in the natural hair journey is most often the first one: actually deciding to go natural. Since Madam C. J. Walker picked up that first hot comb in the early 1900s, black women have been building culture around hair. And we hesitate to step outside of what we've grown up with. We fear that our loved ones won't support our decision, that we'll regret our big chop, that we'll miss our relaxers, that our significant other will hate our new do, that we won't be able to pull off natural hair, and that we won't be able to take care of it.

big chop \'big 'chäp\

[noun, verb]
Cutting off all your chemically treated hair in one fell swoop. Some women do it themselves. Others have a significant other, family member, or barber do it.

We won't insult you by dismissing these fears as myths. They are all valid fears, and for many of us—even those of us who never had a relaxer but developed a flat-iron dependency—this makes going natural one of the bravest things we will ever do. Going natural means facing many of our fears. It also means standing up for ourselves and learning a new skill set.

But if you've ever faced your fears head-on, you already know how wonderful it feels after you've vanquished them. Make no mistake: going natural will require a full-on hair fear confrontation. You might also have to learn to deal with negative comments and to take care of your hair from scratch. But here are three pieces of good news: (1) You *can* do it. (2) We can help you. (3) You're going to come out of this transition looking *amazing*.

So let's get started.

Though many curlfriends refer to getting rid of their relaxed or locked hair as *the big chop,* there is more than one way to go about big chopping.

THE SPONTANEOUS BIG CHOP

A favorite move of college students, artists, movie characters, and New Year's resoluters the world over, spontaneous big choppers cut their hair within a few days or weeks of deciding to go natural.

I was looking at my bank account, and I had to get my ends done, but I only had, like, fifty bucks to get me through to the end of the month, so I walked into a barber shop and told them to cut it all off. It only cost fifteen dollars. —Rhonda

I had some heat damage, and I wasn't pleased. Also, I felt that hair held on to a lot of energy, and 2010 was a rough year. So I decided to chop it all off. My mom cut my hair. —Cassie

My hair and I just didn't get along—it was always frizzy, and I was tired of straightening it every day on top of getting relaxers. It wouldn't stay straight; it wouldn't hold a curl. That's when I realized I was ready to get rid of it. I wasn't thinking about going natural, I just wanted to get rid of that stupid hair. I was twenty-one, a junior in college, and very spontaneous. —Khalia

I only transitioned for about two and a half months due to damage and breakage at the line of demarcation. My natural and relaxed hair were not playing nicely together! —Song Bird

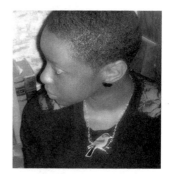

I decided to have a barber cut my hair in January 2011 after realizing I wanted to save some money and was tired of sweating out perms at the gym.

—CHARNELE ASHLEE

when you're forced to big chop for health reasons

Even those who have the luxury of taking the time to research and learn about the beauty and versatility of natural hair may still have hesitations and have to deal with confidence issues. So being forced into a short haircut and learning to work with your natural texture can feel daunting and overwhelming. Do your research, just as you would have if you chose to big chop on your own. Find support in your community and online, find pictures of women with gorgeous short haircuts in magazines and online, and take things slowly. If you're truly uncomfortable, don a wig and ease into your natural hair more gradually. It's a huge step to take, and it can be a difficult one if you aren't able to do the upfront prep work involved with a slower transition. Remember that the way we feel about ourselves plays into our health, too. It's all connected. If you experience depression or anxiety, it may not be a bad idea to see a therapist about it. People can grieve for their hair, especially if it is a big part of their image. Don't be afraid to reach out for as much help as you need with this sudden transition. For more tips on how to manage your new style, go to chapter 2.

None of my transition styles held up well in humidity. My permed hair turned against me and started to fall out. Frustrated, I said, "Let's do this." —Dominique

There are a few reasons to opt for a spontaneous big chop. Some women love adventure and would rather begin their natural hair journey sooner than later. Some women would rather not deal with the gradual transitioning process. And some women are forced into a spontaneous big chop for health reasons (see Nikki's Therapy Corner on page 10).

But be forewarned, while there is no universal right or wrong time to big chop, even the most adventurous woman must feel ready before cutting. Women who take more than a few weeks to transition are more likely to be happy with their decision to go natural and are also more likely to stay natural. Although it can be fun to do a spontaneous chop, most of us will feel more comfortable with a medium to long-term transition. Think about the last time you went to the mall and made a spontaneous purchase that put a huge dent on your credit card. If you cried all the way home, you might want to consider long-term transitioning.

TRANSITIONING

If you want to stay with your hairdresser while transitioning, that is totally fine. Many women employ weaves, extensions, braids, or wigs during the transition period. You can also get through this period on your own. In fact, there's no better way to slowly let go of your relaxer while getting to know your new hair.

The *spontaneous chopper*, as described in the preceding pages, often has to scramble to learn how to take care of her hair in its new short and natural state. As a result, many spontaneous choppers eventually give up on natural hair after a few months, because the learning curve is just too steep. In contrast, a *transitioner* has the chance to practice many of the styles she'll be wearing when she's completely natural. While

spontaneous chops are a great adventure, if you want to stick
with natural hair for the long term, it might be best to transition slowly into becoming a natural.

Many women big chop after six to twenty-four months of
transitioning. But some women wait even longer. Don't let anyone pressure you. You'll know when you're ready to big chop, if
at all. Have faith in your instincts.

While you're transitioning, you'll have to manage two
very different hair textures: your relaxed hair and your natural new growth. Your transition time often depends less on
how long you want your hair to be and more on how long you're
willing to deal with this potentially frustrating hair situation.

The line of demarcation, or the line at which the two different textures meet, is very fragile and prone to matting and
tangling. (Think of the line of demarcation as that awkward
moment when your old friends from high school met your new
friends from college for the first time.) Here are three styles
that blend your two textures.

Rollersets

Rollersets mask the two textures, allow you to show length, and can act as a primer for a beautiful updo.

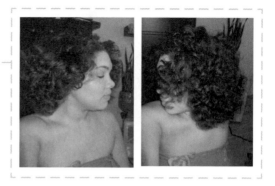

STEP 1 Apply a lightweight leave-in conditioner to your cleansed and conditioned damp hair.

STEP 2 Finger-part the hair into sections, apply a little setting lotion, smooth through, and wrap the hair around a roller and secure it with a pin or a clip. (If you want looser curls, like those pictured, choose large magnetic rollers. For tighter curls and waves, opt for small magnetic rollers or flexi rods.)

STEP 3 Allow the hair to air dry or sit under a dryer until your hair is completely dry. *Taking down the rollers prematurely will result in a very frizzy set!*

STEP 4 Finger-style and go!

Fancy Faux Bun

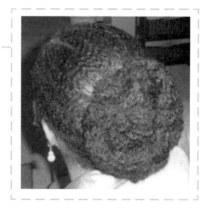

Smooth wet or dry hair into a ponytail using your hands and a boar bristle brush to smooth the edges if necessary. Apply a bit of shea butter to your edges and tie on a silk scarf to allow the hair to set. Next, pop on a fake bun in the back (purchased at your local beauty-supply store to match your hair color and texture), and there ya go!

Fierce Braid-and-Curl

This is one of those styles that work when you're transitioning and *really* work when you get past the teeny weeny afro stage. A fluffy elongated braid-out is best done on freshly cleansed hair.

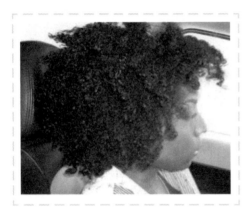

STEP 1 Gently blow out your damp hair using a blow-dryer. Be sure to apply a heat protectant first as well as a light leave-in conditioner. In this case, use the tension method, in which you gently stretch the hair with one hand while applying heat from the dryer with the other. (This method is less stressful than using a comb attachment or a round or paddle brush.) Keep the heat to a minimum and keep the dryer six inches from your hair. Also, remember to angle the blow-dryer downward.

STEP 2 Once the hair is blown out, divide the hair into sections and braid each section, remembering that the smaller the braids, the tighter the wave pattern. Aim for around ten to twelve braids, and use an oil or pomade on each section before you start braiding.

STEP 3 For added texture, roll the last two inches of each braid on a small satin-covered roller.

STEP 4 Let your hair set overnight, then unbraid it to reveal beautiful waves and curls in the morning.

THE ACTUAL BIG CHOP

While transitioning, you've played with your hair, you've gotten to know it, and you're finally ready to commit to being natural. Now what?

First, consider what you want your hair to look like after you big chop.

If you want to start out with a simple teeny weeny afro (TWA), then a significant other or family member can do the job for you with an electric razor. As we'll discuss later, this is a great way to make a loved one feel like he or she is taking part in your natural hair journey.

However, if you want a more complicated hairstyle, it's a good idea to go to a barber or a hairstylist for your big chop. But don't just hit the Internet for recommendations or walk into the first barbershop or natural hair care salon you find. Ask your natural friends for referrals, and while you're at it, ask them about their own big chop experiences. Remember, every curlie has a story to tell, and your friends who are already natural can be a great source of inspiration, warnings, and advice. If all else fails, hit the CurlyNikki forums and ask other naturals in your area for suggestions.

Once you've settled on a hairstylist, make an appointment at a time that leaves you at least a few hours to get used to the new do before you have to socialize with others. Also take the time to find pictures of women whose hair you'd like to emulate. Print or cut those pictures out and bring them along with you to your appointment so that both you and the person cutting your hair have a physical touchstone for the look you're

If You Decide to Go Natural with a Hairstylist

By Marie Simone

If you're thinking about going natural, it's important to keep a few things in mind to make sure you enjoy a successful transition.

* **EDUCATE YOURSELF.** Talk to friends and family members who wear their hair natural and find out more about their experience. You should also read blogs such as CurlyNikki, watch credible natural hair videos, and read hair magazines to find out what's really involved in making the transition to natural hair. And don't forget that you know your own hair better than anybody. Get familiar with your hair texture and wave pattern. If you're not sure about it, talk with a licensed hairstylist.

* **CONSULT WITH A HAIRSTYLIST WHO REALLY KNOWS ABOUT NATURAL HAIR.** Just because people are hairstylists doesn't mean they are skilled in styling and maintaining *natural* hair. I find that many stylists have been told that natural hair is harder to do, needs more products, and dries out easily. But remember, hair is hair; you just have to take care of natural hair differently. When you have your consultation with a potential natural hairstylist, prepare a checklist and ask the following questions:

    * What kind of texture do I have?
    * Is my hair dry or oily?
    * Is my hair coarse, medium, or fine?
    * Does my hair absorb moisture?

- What kind of curl pattern do I have?
- Do I have the same curl pattern throughout my hair or does it vary?
- What natural hairstyle would work best for me?
- What steps will I need to take to maintain it?

Make sure he or she touches and feels your hair to answer these questions accurately. Also, be patient with a stylist who may not be familiar with your hair. He or she will need time to really understand your hair texture. Sometimes your hair can read one way to the touch but after shampooing can read differently.

* **MAKE YOUR CHOICE.** Don't be coerced into going natural simply because people you know are making the change and suggest that you do the same. Once you educate yourself, you have to look at your own lifestyle and decide what kind of maintenance routine works best for you. Think about the time you *need* versus the time you *have* to maintain your hair as well as the products you're willing to use and pay for. You should consider all of these factors when making your final decision.

* **STICK WITH IT.** It's common to see people begin the transition to natural hair and then change their mind and go back to relaxed hair—and then change their mind again. If I have clients who've started to switch to natural hair and are thinking about giving up on it, my first question to them is why. Some people feel that they don't have time to maintain their hair. Others get discouraged because they aren't sure how to handle situations such as the effect of moisture or summertime heat on their natural hair. But those issues can be addressed with the right information and products. Sure, there are cases when some people conclude that natural hair just isn't for them. But usually, with the right resources and tools, most clients continue to go forward with their transition successfully. Natural hair is like anything else in life: if you want to get sharper at it and understand it more, you have to continue to educate yourself. It's a journey, and you have to have patience.

* **HAVE FUN.** A lot of people try to put natural hair in a box or turn it into a formula. But I encourage people who wear natural hair to play with it and to stay open to new styles and techniques. The beauty of natural hair is its versatility. You can twist it and take it down; twist it, put it in a ball, and take it down; twist and roll the ends and take it down. Don't get in a rut and think that there are only a few things you can do with natural hair. In its natural state, your hair has endless possibilities. So be free, go with the flow, and embrace your natural texture. And most of all, have fun!

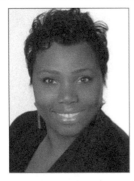

Marie Simone's work has been featured in top hair, fashion, and lifestyle magazines, including *Modern Salon*, *Essence*, *Behind the Chair*, *Sophisticate's Black Hair*, and *InStyle*. Other credits include assisting for Fashion Week New York's Number:Lab Men's Show; a salon showcase on the reality television series *Split Ends*; instructional video appearances, including *What's Hot in My Salon*; work as an onset commercial hairstylist for Dark and Lovely; and appearances on the natural hair blog CurlyNikki.com.

going for. A lot can get lost in translation when you're describing what you want, and a picture can save the day.

AFTER THE BIG CHOP

When we talk about being scared of the big chop, what we're really talking about is being scared of what will happen *after* the big chop. We'll address three of the biggest fears here:

Reason 1:
I won't be able to take care of it.

Yes, you will. Keep reading; we'll show you how.

Reason 2:
My significant other might hate it.

Contrary to popular belief, many men prefer natural hairstyles. "When my husband and I met twelve years ago, a big part of the initial attraction for him was the fact that I was natural. He's just not a fan of bone straight hair, whether chemically induced or achieved with heat on natural hair," says one curlfriend.

Some men, like Nikki's hubby, even wage campaigns to get their significant others to go natural. Another curlfriend told us, "My husband loves [my hair]. He encouraged me to go natural and he certainly loves the money I'm saving by not going to the hairdresser every two weeks. He thinks all African American women should wear their natural hair. He hasn't seen a head of natural, healthy-looking hair he didn't like."

However, going natural can and has become an issue in many a black woman's relationship. We've heard of curlies whose boyfriends are constantly nagging them to go back to straight hair. And in a few (very rare) cases, curlfriends have been dumped over this issue.

After decades of seeing straight and superstraight hair as the beauty standard for black women, some men might respond poorly to your decision to go natural, which puts you in a difficult position. On one hand, you don't want your man "up in your hair." On the other hand, you don't want him to find you less attractive because you've decided to switch to natural hair.

Some of you might be tempted to surprise your significant other with your big chop. You figure it's your hair and you don't need his permission, so you go from relaxed to natural without telling him first. Even though we understand the reasoning behind this move, we don't endorse it. By going behind his back, you might end up missing an opportunity to take (as opposed to drag) your man along on your natural hair journey.

Here are five tips for transitioning your man to accept your decision to go natural.

1. HAVE AN OPEN DISCUSSION ABOUT IT. Introduce him to the idea; let him know why you've decided to big chop or transition. He needs to understand that you're not just springing this on him and that you respect his opinions and feelings, but at the end of the day, it's your head.

2. INTRODUCE HIM TO THE ONLINE NATURAL HAIR WORLD.
   Show him the research on how damaging relaxers
   can be and what a fantastic alternative natural hair
   is. Show him the support that exists and the vast
   numbers of other women who have decided to go
   natural. Let him know that he won't be the only guy
   on the block with a natural partner.

3. EXPLAIN THE VERSATILITY YOU'LL ENJOY WITH
   NATURAL HAIR. Show him pictures of natural
   women with straight hair, curly hair, highly curly
   hair, wavy hair, buns, ponytails, puffs, afros,
   braids, twists, and so on. Natural is not just one
   look. Men can be visual creatures; show him lots
   of pictures and examples.

4. KNOW THAT IT MAY TAKE HIM SOME TIME TO WARM UP
   TO THE IDEA. It's a process and you shouldn't get
   angry with him if he's not jazzed on the spot about
   you going natural. Let it marinate a bit, giving him
   the chance to process it all.

5. BE CONFIDENT! If you're exuding happiness and
   confidence, he can't help but support you.

Reason 3:
My mom might hate it!

Many of us were raised by mothers who welcomed the advance
of the relaxer with open arms. They tell us horror stories about
conks* and hot combs that had to be heated with real fire on

---

* Popular during the 1920s through the 1960s, a conk was an early gel form of
  the relaxer, most notable for its main ingredient, a harsh lye, which made its
  application particularly painful.

My Mom *Hated* My Hair!

By Chatel Theagene from *Back to Curly*

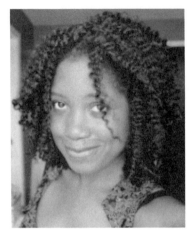

Doing the big chop is oftentimes a newly natural's least favorite part of the natural hair journey for reasons that seem to manifest themselves with each backhanded compliment thrown her way. Many choose to transition for longer periods of time in order to avoid bewildered stares from our loved ones and friends. But for those who are on the road to the big chop and are regularly subject to the misperceptions and ignorance of others, take heart in the fact that you are not alone.

Today it's remarkably easy to look back and regard with new understanding the judgments from most of my family. There were *many*, but none more complex and sordid than that of my own mother. My first big chop over ten years ago shook up my mother something awful: the cold shoulders and questioning eyes followed me around for months. For a Caribbean mother, hair—*long* hair at that—is your saving grace, your accessory du jour if ever you forget to wear your favorite earrings or necklace.

There was disappointment and fear written across my mother's face, and yet my decision to big chop was something for which I could not rightfully apologize. At eighteen, I was taking on a new identity and my outlook on life was similar to many of my peers', and doing the big chop felt right. Why apologize for coming into your own, no matter what path you choose? This was my first lesson.

I talked to her as any young woman would talk to her mother and allowed her the space to get to her kind of normal. I'd already reached mine. Her perceptions based on my decision to go natural remained just that—her own. And over time she came to accept my hair.

There's no momentous white flag to inform you of this acceptance, but hindsight will send you proof. Your loved ones will still love you and will still care for and accept you, even if they don't understand your decision to go natural. That is their own journey to take.

Years later my mother was able to embark on her own natural hair journey. Ironically, today we gossip over the phone about hair regimens, products she's trying, hair creams I love, and at-home mixes that are incredibly easy to make!

We all greatly inspire both our doubters and our mothers, even if we cannot see it right after our big chop. Stepping out on faith and loving the journey regardless of the detractors and naysayers are what solidify any person's decision to be who they truly are.

- -

Chatel Theagene, aka "Chai," is a writer, natural hair enthusiast, and foodie based in the trenches of Brooklyn, New York. Find her musings over at the blog *Back to Curly*, where she celebrates all things natural hair, life, and love.

real stoves. And our grandmothers wear wigs. Not only has natural hair care not been passed down through the generations, many curlfriends report that their mothers go buck wild when their daughters decide to big chop.

To be fair, we've heard many heartwarming stories about mothers being nothing but supportive of their daughters' decision to go natural. But we've also heard of mothers crying, mothers screaming, and mothers predicting that their daughters have *ruined* their lives and any chance at love or career success that they might have had, all because they've abandoned their relaxers.

And this reaction can get even more extreme if you decide to go the TWA route. One of our curlfriends told us this story: "My mother has issues with long hair. She loves it and will hang on to it even if her hair is damaged. When I first went natural, I decided to cut off all my hair. My mother had no problem with me going natural, as she herself was natural for many years, getting a press and curl. But when I cut my hair off, my mother thought that I had lost my mind! She thought I was having a nervous breakdown and literally got on her hands and knees to pray for me, as she thought I was losing it."

We tell you this not to scare you but to prepare you. Your mother may be supportive, but she also might say hurtful things that cause you to feel like "Cindercurly," stuck at home washing the hot combs, questioning your beauty and your decision to go natural.

Let us just say this right now: you are beautiful, no matter if your hair is natural or relaxed. If people try to tell you otherwise, they do so because of their own issues. Remember, these insults say more about them than they do about you.

We hope the following tips will help you when dealing with negative comments from loved ones after your big chop.

1. TALK TO YOUR FAMILY. Try to have a calm, rational discussion with them about your decision (even if they're going off the handle).

2. SHOW THEM HOW BEAUTIFUL AND VERSATILE NATURAL HAIR IS (PICTURES IN MAGAZINES, ONLINE, ETC.). For example, if they claim you won't be able to get a job with natural hair, show them a picture of Ursula Burns, the CEO of Xerox, the first black female CEO of a Fortune 500 company and a proud TWA wearer.

3. HAVE SOME QUICK, WITTY COMEBACKS ON HAND FOR THE OCCASIONAL SNARKY COMMENT. "What are you going to do with your hair?" Response: "What are you going to do with yours?"

4. GIVE THEM SPACE AND TIME TO GET USED TO THE IDEA. Respect their feelings and opinions as you have asked them to respect yours. Time has a way of fixing most things.

5. EXUDE CONFIDENCE. Smile and hold your head up high, even when you're not feeling confident. Before you ask them to accept you, you must accept yourself. Oh, and if you must, fake it till you make it!

Of all these tips, number five is the most important. Confidence is engaging and contagious. Time and time again, we've heard stories of family members responding badly to a big chop, only to turn around and go natural themselves, when they see how happy and confident their natural relative is. Remember the mom who dropped to her knees and *prayed* for her daughter after she came home with a TWA? She went on to do a big chop of her own.

So when your loved ones are giving you grief, just remember that even your fiercest detractors might end up asking you for transition and natural hair tips by this time next year. Do us a favor when they do. Buy them a copy of this book.

TIPS FOR TERRIFIC TRANSITIONING

* Remember, THERE IS NO WRONG OR RIGHT WAY TO TRANSITION.
* The LINE OF DEMARCATION where the relaxed hair ends and the new growth starts is very delicate. Please treat your hair like silk until you are ready to do the big chop.
* CONDITIONER-WASH (CO-WASH) YOUR HAIR at least once a week to add moisture to your hair. If you are not ready to co-wash only, then wash your hair with diluted shampoo followed by a conditioner. (We'll cover both of these processes in the next chapter.)
* BIG CHOP WHEN YOU ARE READY. Don't cut your hair until you are emotionally prepared.
* DEEP CONDITION your hair at least once a week. Check out our deep condition product suggestions at the back of the book.
* BE VERY CAREFUL WHEN USING HEAT ON YOUR HAIR.

You could potentially damage your healthy new growth by flat-ironing, hot curling, or blow-drying your hair too often.

* CONCENTRATE ON YOUR OWN HAIR, NOT YOUR NEIGHBOR'S. Naturally curly hair is unique and varies from person to person. Sometimes your hair type looks completely different once you cut your hair. Don't be discouraged. This is the hair God gave you, so therefore it is beautiful.

* START TAKING MONTHLY PICTURES. This will help you chart your progress and give you a confidence boost on those days when you think your hair is not growing quickly enough. Look how far you've come!

* WRITE IN A JOURNAL OR START A BLOG. It will help you keep things in perspective. Before you reach for the relaxer or make an appointment for a Brazilian blowout, try to remember why you wanted to transition in the first place.

* JOIN THE CURLYNIKKI FORUMS. Your online hair community is waiting for you, and we'll provide you with so much encouragement and advice, you'll wonder how you ever got along without us.

YOUR TRANSITION ROUTINE GUIDE

Daily Routine

Keep your hair lubricated and/or protected. Apply a little water and a water-based moisturizer to the ends and seal with

Will a Natural Hairstyle Hold Your Career Back? *No!*

By Monique King-Viehland

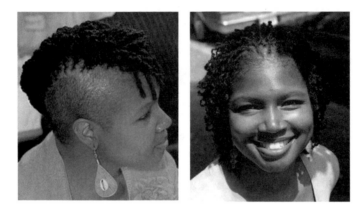

I have been doing real estate and economic development for more than a decade. In the hundreds of meetings I have attended over the last ten years, I have typically been the only woman, the only person of color, and the youngest person in the room. And if that isn't enough to make my new business acquaintances do a double take, I rock ethnocentric jewelry and locs.

My hair has been natural for about fourteen years. I started my natural hair journey well before I graduated with my master's degree in 2001 and headed into the working world. First, it was a short TWA, which I dyed blond for a while. After that I gave up the dye and shaved my hair pretty close to the scalp and wore it that way for nearly eight years. Then in 2006, I decided to lock my hair and haven't looked back.

Throughout my career, I have been responsible for multimillion-dollar projects, obtained millions of dollars in project funding, and consistently advanced in my field; my salary has increased 205 percent since I started. Today I am the president of a for-profit development corporation, and I broke ground on an $80 million project last year.

I am sure there are sisters out there who would say that natural hair is frowned upon in the professional world, but I haven't found that to be true at all. I can honestly say that my natural hair has never been an impediment to being successful in my career—even though my chosen field is predominantly white and male.

Moreover, I have several friends and colleagues rocking naturals in conservative offices all across the United States. Several of my natural friends from college and graduate school have gone on to become successful lawyers, doctors, investment bankers, and business executives, and their hair didn't hold them back at all. If you're not advancing in your career or you don't get that job you interviewed for, look to other factors. Blaming your hair might lead you to overlook other possible issues that are holding you back.

Throughout my career, my natural hair has been a huge part of who I am, but it has never been more important to my bosses, colleagues, and clients than how well I do my job. So even if they do a double take when I walk in the room, once I open my mouth, they realize that this woman knows her stuff. At the end of the day, that is what matters most to them and to me.

Monique King-Viehland has served as executive director of the Capital City Redevelopment Association for the State of New Jersey. In 2004 she was named one of *Pittsburgh Magazine*'s "40 under 40," and in 2008 her story was featured in the book *What I Know Now: Letters to My Younger Self*, along with pieces on Maya Angelou and Cokie Roberts. She is currently president of the Campus Gateway Development Corporation at NJIT, where she oversees several multimillion-dollar projects. She has been natural since the age of twenty, and it has never held her back.

a hair oil. Wear your hair in protective or low-manipulation styles such as buns and wet sets (styles you do while your hair is wet). Try not to comb your hair daily if it can be avoided; use your fingers as your primary styling tool.

Nightly Routine

Remove any pins, tight ponytail holders, and other hair accessories before going to bed. Secure your hair (twists, braids, a loose bun, etc.) and cover your head with a satin bonnet. If you have problems keeping a satin bonnet on at night, try sleeping on a satin pillowcase. Remoisturize your hair if it feels dry and its texture brings to mind a haystack.

Weekly Routine

STEP 1 Using your fingers, gently detangle your hair to prep it for washing. If your hair is particularly dry, you can do an oil treatment before washing. Simply add oil to your dry hair, put on a plastic cap, and wait for 15 to 30 minutes while your body heat allows the oil to penetrate the hair shaft.

STEP 2 Cleanse your hair with a mild (sulfate-free) shampoo, ideally in the shower.

STEP 3 Follow cleansing with a moisturizing conditioner. Detangle your hair under the water stream with a wide tooth comb and/or your fingers. (We cover detangling more extensively in chapter 3.)

STEP 4 Rinse the conditioner out of your hair, blot your hair dry, and apply a deep conditioner.

STEP 5 Put on a plastic cap and sit under a warm dryer for 15 to 30 minutes. This is a great time to look at the styles we cover later in the book, many of which can be used on transitioning hair.

STEP 6 Get back in the shower, rinse out the deep conditioner, and blot your hair dry.

STEP 7 Style as preferred, but we recommend wet sets.

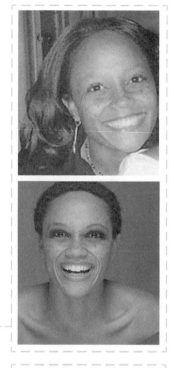

BIG CHOPPERS SOUND OFF!

I'm so impressed that I choose to present my natural hair to the world. I just feel good about it, especially when most of the women around me have relaxed hair. I was such a hair-confident person when my hair was relaxed (my hair is naturally an auburn color and was fairly long). I didn't realize how much of my personal idea of beauty had to do with how I felt about my hair. So now that it's all cut off and all natural, I'm proud that I still feel beautiful—even more so because I'm wearing my hair natural.

—Autumn

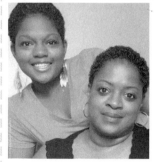

When I decided to go natural roughly two years ago, my daughter was very supportive but made it clear that was my thing, not hers. She kept her hair short but would not give up the "creamy crack." I would inform but never criticize. So imagine my joy when she posted on Facebook that she wanted to cut off her hair and go natural. We made the appointment and the rest is history.

—Gaye (pictured with her daughter)

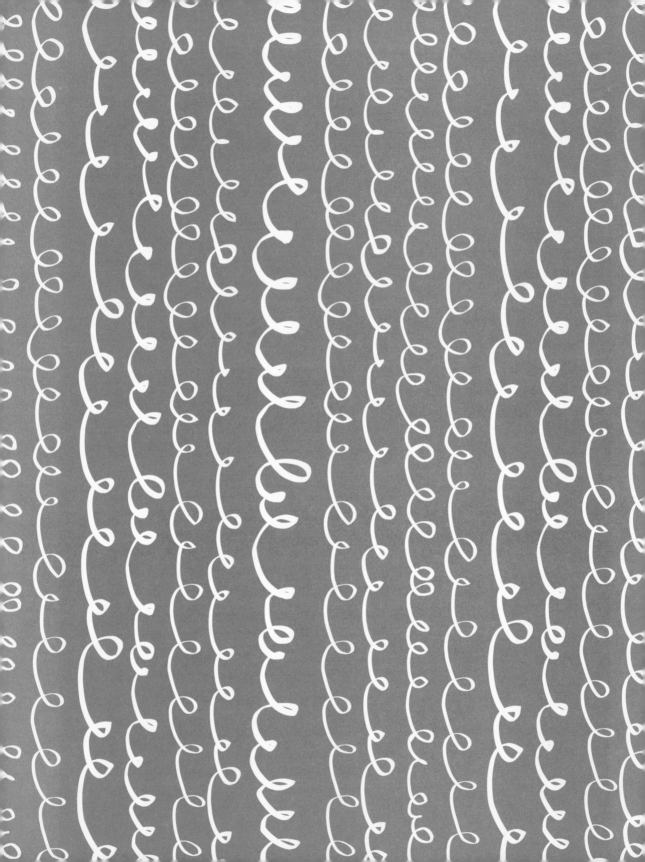

CHAPTER TWO

TWA

How to Nurture Your Teeny Weeny Afro

Many women start their natural hair journey with what we in the curly community affectionately call a teeny weeny afro (TWA). In this chapter, we'll discuss how to form a relationship with your new hairstyle, and give practical and emotional advice for looking and feeling feminine with short hair.

To the readers who are skimming this book, this is the chapter you'll want to read thoroughly. Although some women have the patience and determination to deal with long transitions, many others choose to cut off all of their hair either spontaneously or after a short transition. If you don't have the patience or desire for a longer transition, know that it's fairly rare for a woman to big chop without having to go through the teeny weeny afro stage. So consider this your preview of what will come if you decide to go natural and big chop.

To the readers who have already big chopped, let us first say, "Congratulations!" You've worked up the courage or simply decided to go with your instinct, or maybe you just got sick of spending hours at the hairdresser. It doesn't matter how you got here, the fact is that you've taken the first big step in your natural hair journey, and there are a few ways you might be feeling about that right now.

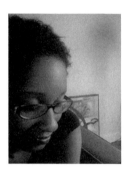

As soon as the last snip was done, I cried for three seconds. It was a release cry. Then I started jumping up and down. I loved it immediately and couldn't believe it. I was seeing the real me after so many years.

—EBONY JOY WILKINS

EXHILARATED: Many of our curlfriends have reported looking into the mirror after cutting their hair and experiencing a huge serotonin spike. They're filled with confidence and joy, and they can now see clearly both their inner and outer beauty. Getting the big chop ain't church, but we've heard of women jumping up and down, dancing, you name it. This is also the time when product junkies pass around the collection plate!

We've even seen women take to YouTube to literally sing the praises of their newly shorn hair. Seriously, if we could bottle this feeling, which can last anywhere from hours to weeks, we'd be billionaires. This is the reaction we hope for for you, but beware, there are other reactions, too.

RELIEVED: It's as if you didn't realize how much your hair had been holding you back or how much it weighed you down until you got rid of it. Many of our curlfriends report feeling lighter and a profound sense of relief after their big chop. For some, hair can carry both spiritual and literal weight, and when it goes away, so do the emotions and problems it carried with it. Also, if you've been transitioning for a while, it sometimes comes as a relief to just get the big chop over with already. Reanell Frederick (pictured in the sidebar on page 64) originally planned to transition into the fall, but by the spring she had grown sick of dealing with two different hair textures. She had to spend twenty minutes arguing with her stylist to agree to big chop her hair earlier than planned, but Reanell has not regretted her decision: "All I thought was, 'Phew, I finally did it!' I felt relieved. I wasn't nervous at all. I was very pleased with the outcome."

UNCOMFORTABLE: Not everyone is exhilarated or relieved after their initial big chop. Quite a few transitioners have found themselves feeling awkward with their new hairdo. It's not that you hate the way you look; it's more like you're not used to it. It's a bit like being assigned a college roommate, someone you've never met before and don't really know yet. This "living with a stranger" feeling has been enough to send a few of our curlfriends back to the creamy crack within just a few months of their big chop.

If you haven't been natural since your single-digit years, it might take a while to get used to this new version of yourself. Just know that much like a rooming assignment between two ultimately compatible people, it doesn't stay awkward for long. You don't have to love your hair from the get-go. Be patient with yourself and your TWA. Give yourself time—at least a year—to fall in love with your new look. Keep in mind that many of the women who return to perms or weaves eventually end up big chopping all over again, this time with their eyes wide open.

OH CRAP! WHAT DID I JUST DO??? Don't worry, this isn't a common reaction after a big chop, but it does happen. Much like the woman who is uncomfortable with her new hairdo, some people just out-and-out hate themselves with short hair. Sometimes people don't realize how much of their look is actually dependent on hair until they get rid of it.

We're not going to lie to you, TWAs are very face-centric. Once you get one, it's like "Bam! Face! Face! Face!" Your mug becomes the main focus on your entire body, and it can be hard on folks who aren't used to face-centered attention. You've heard the phrase "Oh, that style really brings out your face." Well, the TWA shoves your face into the spotlight, which can dredge up a lot of beauty issues, and your initial response to short hair can end up being, "Oh crap! What did I do? I've *ruined* my looks with this hairstyle. And I look like a boy."

But don't worry, and don't rush out to get a wig. We're here to help. Meet us in the next section.

The Beauty of Being Bald

By Leandra Williams

I immediately mourned the loss of my hair, even as I was cutting it. "I just don't think I'm cute enough to pull this off," I told my sister. Despite the many compliments tossed my way—"I love it!" "Leandra?! You look stunning"—I felt pretty insecure. Before, I had my face plus really cool hair. Now, I just had my face. Initially, I wore more makeup than usual. I would say, "I don't want to look like a little boy," but really I just didn't think I was attractive enough to successfully be without hair. I wanted to look in the mirror and know instantly, *"This is me."* I didn't.

What I *did* know was that I was about to become really familiar with my face. And although I was uncomfortable, I knew I had to settle into the discomfort and feel it out. Really, what other choice do you have when you shave your head? It'll grow back, yes, but it takes time. In the meantime, you can attempt to overcompensate or you can decide to get comfortable. I chose the latter.

I've returned to wearing my usual amount of makeup, which consists of mascara and maybe subtle eye shadow and/or eyeliner. The darker my hair got, the more I liked it, and while I still have not yet felt the "This is me" feeling, I know I'm getting there without developing any more complexes regarding my looks.

If you've recently cut your hair or plan to do so soon, realize the opportunity it presents to you to love yourself even more. It's a reawakening. A new beginning of sorts, and an opportunity to connect to yourself, to your beauty, and to your people.

Leandra Williams writes about the lessons she's learned in her attempts to transform herself and her life into her highest vision on the blog *What My World's Like*. Armed with a sunny spirit and a warm smile, she lives off of laughter, love, and music. She can be found in Brooklyn, New York, finding the good and being inspired.

THE ISSUES THAT COME UP WITH TWAs

Oh my gosh, I look like a boy—or even worse, a man.

Listen, some women are just delicate of face. They get a short do, and they come out looking like a pixie. If that's you, awesome. But for the rest of us, short hair might make us feel a little unfeminine. The good news is that "feminine" is often just a little bit of research and a few shopping trips away. Here's what every woman should do as soon as she big chops.

1. GO ON AN EARRING SPREE. After you get your big chop, we suggest immediately hitting the nearest cheap earring store. Use the money you're saving on hair appointments to buy at least $50 worth of earrings in all shapes and sizes—though we say the bigger, the better. Don't limit yourself to the earrings you would have worn with longer hair. The magic of a shorter cut is that you can pull off all sorts of looks you couldn't before—so take advantage. The right pair of earrings will take you from boyish to kapow!

2. BUY HEADBANDS, BOWS, AND FLOWERS. We just about proselytize for headbands, bows, and flowers at CurlyNikki.com. You'd seriously think we had stock in the website Etsy. We don't, but we have found these three things to be transformative. Put

I was never a fan of big or dangling earrings because my hair was longer and was the best accessory. Now, I'm a sucker for them. My makeup is the same as before I cut my hair, except that I use bolder colors now. I feel I can do this now because my face takes center stage instead of my hair, so the bolder colors don't clash.

—KIMBERLY HAWTHORNE

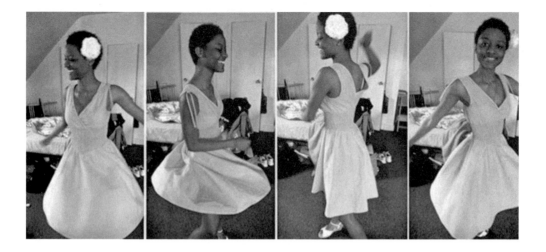

on a pretty little A-line dress and an even prettier flower headband, and trust us, no one will mistake you for a boy.

3. FIND PICTURES OF WOMEN WITH A SIMILAR FACIAL SHAPE TO YOURS. Go to sites such as CurlyNikki.com and YouTube to see pictures of women with similar facial shapes rocking their TWAs. See how they fem up, and take notes.

4. REASSESS YOUR WARDROBE. In our opinion, the most interesting side effect of going natural is that you can suddenly pull off all sorts of looks you weren't able to rock before. This means that the woman who used to look good only in outfits purchased from J. Crew and Banana Republic can now handle an edgier punk-rock off-the-shoulder top on weekends or go full-on vintage glam for her cousin's wedding.

TWAs are very versatile and go with a ton of different looks—except for sweats. Wear sweats with a TWA and risk looking like a freshman point guard for a boys' basketball team. You can get rid

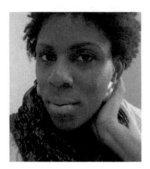

I always wore
earrings and
jewelry when I
was relaxed. That
hasn't changed,
but now I wear a
bit more makeup.
Being natural
has boosted my
confidence. I find
myself dressing
edgier and taking
more risks. I
wear a watch,
some bangles, and
earrings. I've also
been experimenting
with different
shades of lipstick
and lip gloss.

— ONYEKA OF
OMALICHACURLS.COM

of all the sloppy stuff in your closet (sweats, male-cut T-shirts, nylon jogging suits, etc.), which tends to look bad with TWAs, and use your new do as an excuse to glam up your wardrobe.

5. LEARN HOW TO DO MAKEUP. Head to the nearest makeup counter (we love MAC) and ask for a tutorial. You can also jump on YouTube or your favorite makeup blog and get creative. Have fun!

A lot of our curlfriends talk about short hair in terms of freedom. They say, "Oh, it allows me more time to do other things" or "I'm not so attached to the way I look anymore." After years of weekly, biweekly, or monthly hair appointments, many women really like not having to deal with so much hair. Some women like this freedom so much that they don't even want to bother with the grow-out process. They'll spend no more than fifteen minutes on their hair daily, they'll rock their accessories, and they'll wonder for the rest of their lives why they didn't get rid of all that pesky hair sooner. If that's you, congratulations on finding your perfect look. Feel free to skip ahead to the styling section.

But for the rest of us, let's delve into some more issues that will probably come up at the beginning of your natural hair journey.

Confidence

We mentioned confidence a lot in chapter 1 on transitioning, and that's because going natural isn't for the faint of heart. Some days you'll receive compliments from strangers on the street. Other days people you hold dear will insult your hair straight to your face. Yes, the compliments are very nice, but man, do those insults sting.

However, at the end of the day, the person whose opinion matters the most is you.

Let us repeat that because it's not something we hear often. As women, we want our looks to please our significant others, we want our family members to respect us, and we just adore admiring glances from strangers. Nonetheless, when it comes to your hair, the person whose opinion matters the most is you.

If you're not already an A+ student in the self-confidence department, don't worry. You're about to become one (get your curly notebooks out!). TWAs have a way of bringing out your confidence. Having one forces you to defend your decisions and stand by your choices. You'll no longer be able to hide behind long hair. A TWA forces you to let your personality shine.

So, yes, fake it until you make it for now, but keep in mind that by the time your TWA has grown out, you'll have way more confidence and probably like yourself even more than when you first began your journey.

Falling in Love

Women make the decision to go natural for many different reasons. And we suggest transitioning as opposed to spontaneously big chopping in the same way we'd suggest getting to know someone for a while before moving in together. A spontaneous chop is moving in after one or two dates. A transition is moving in together after many months or years.

Getting Your Accessories in Order

By Ni-Kiya Alleyne

I understand the depressing feeling you experience the day after you wake up to your short do. When I woke up the morning after my big chop, I was bare-faced and groggy, no earrings—and I had supershort hair. I just stared at myself in the mirror because I was in utter shock. I didn't look like the person I'd become accustomed to waking up to for the last couple of years.

That morning my mother told me I looked like my brother, before giving me a disgusted laugh and walking off. For a split second it affected me; it hurt me. Did I really look like a boy? Crap! I needed to do something! I never ever thought about hiding my hair under weaves, wigs, or hats. I don't believe that after the big chop you should succumb to those measures. I only thought about how I would *rock it.*

I threw all of my accessories on the floor and sat smack-dab in the middle of them, figuring out what would work for me at this stage in my life and what wouldn't. I had chopsticks, ponytail holders, and other hair accessories that, of course, would be of no use to me at this point, so I hid them.

I carefully picked my earrings out of the accessories pile and put them up on display. I also separated my headbands and put them all together. I wanted to make sure I saw my accessories collection every day. I said to myself, "So your hair is too short to do anything with it—*pop* the accessories!"

In my opinion, accessories can change or update any outfit. One person can wear a black shirt and jeans, and with the use of

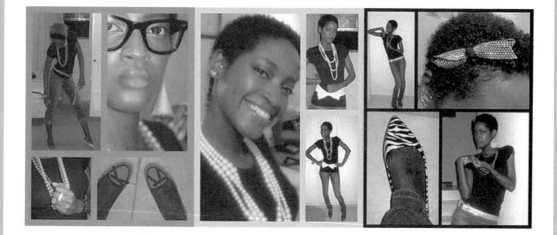

accessories, the outfit can take on a different look each time. Even though I was obsessed with accessories before my big chop—I loved different shoes, belts, earrings, hats, and so forth—I found myself gravitating more to my headbands and earrings to really rock my TWA. Makeup also plays an important role. Not a lot of anything is needed, just enough.

I'm a very funky feeling sort of girl. I like bright colors and odd shapes—anything that can be described as very strange—and my accessories are like that. My sister is very conservative, and it shows in her accessories. Each person is different, so use your accessories to make yourself look feminine, cute, glamorous, chic. Use them to show off your personality. You do not need long hair to feel feminine or to rock a certain look.

But in either case, you'll have to get to know your hair on another level. This is the part that trips up many big choppers. Before their big chop, they imagine going natural as a music video filled with camera-ready looks, perfect products, and a bouncy beat that matches their new attitude. But news flash: the title of this book isn't *Confessions of a Curly Vixen*.

We've been in the natural hair game for a while now, and we've never heard of a completely smooth natural hair journey. Just as you're not going to be 100 percent in love with the person you share a home with every moment of every day, you're not going to love your hair all day every day, either.

You may be surprised that your hair doesn't look exactly like the hair you've seen on the natural beauties in *Essence*

why we don't talk about hair grades

If you've done any online research regarding natural hair, you've probably come across people talking about hair grading: 4C, 3B, 2A—it's hard to keep it all straight. However, in this book, you'll find no references to hair grades. Just lots of great styles and tips for every texture. We feel that grading your hair is a bit like comparing your spouse with Linda's husband. Linda's husband may do this and he might do that, but there are many things that your husband does that Linda's husband doesn't do. It's the same with hair: there's stuff that your hair does that others' hair doesn't (and if anyone has hair that knows how to take out the trash, please forward your name and address to us STAT!). Achieving better than good hair is all about experimenting until you get it right. Grading impedes true experimentation so we won't be using it. We say, give your own hair an A+ and move on from the subject of grades altogether.

brace yourself for natural highs and lows

Every day with your TWA will not be unicorns and rainbows. Some days you'll love your new do. Some days you'll hate it. Looks and mood often intertwine to the detriment of both. Sometimes our outside problems can affect the way we feel about our hair, and sometimes not loving what we see in the mirror that morning can negatively influence the rest of our day. Understand that and keep in mind that your natural hair journey is reflective of your life's journey. There will be ups and downs, hills and valleys. Embrace and appreciate the entire cycle.

magazine or even on the street. When you use a relaxer, you can pretty much take a picture you see in a magazine to your stylist and get that exact same haircut. But realize that natural hair textures vary greatly. Even if you put a lot of effort into grading your hair (which we don't recommend [see the sidebar on page 44]), your hair will not look the same as that glamorous sister's in the YouTube video or even as your own biological sister's, even though she comes from the exact same genetic pool as you.

Here's the hardest part about having natural hair—at least at first: getting to know it. You need to get to know your hair. It really is that simple. Sure, reach out for styling advice, and by all means, gather as many tips as possible. But realize that at the end of the day, it's just you and *your* fro. You will have to get to know it, experiment with it, and, most important, work with what you have, not with what you want.

Nappier Than Expected Syndrome

By LV Burns

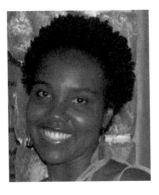 When I first big chopped, my hair was nappier than I expected it to be. Before the big chop, I looked at a lot of hair photos. Looking at some of the curlier, shinier hair textures, I thought, *Maybe my hair will look like that.* I even looked at my childhood (before I had a relaxer) photos and studied my natural texture and thought, *Well, my hair won't be as nappy as it was back then.* However, after I cut out my relaxed hair, I found out that those photos didn't lie.

I think a lot of new naturals experience this. The new growth that you see when your hair is relaxed has been altered by chemicals. It does not necessarily represent what your hair will look like after you big chop, and some people revert back to relaxers after doing the big chop because their hair is nappier than they expected. I call this the Nappier Than Expected Syndrome.

In some cases, Nappier Than Expected Syndrome causes you to go out and search for products that will make your hair curlier and shinier. These products do not work, so you go and buy more. In reality, your hair is most likely not meant to be curlier or shinier. After the products don't work, some of us start thinking, *Maybe I can't do this natural thing.* I want to stop you right there. I am begging you to hang in there. If you do, you're in for a treat.

Nappier Than Expected Syndrome is not a bad thing once you get past the initial shock. When I finally stopped trying to turn my hair into something it's not, I began to let go of the notion that my hair should be less nappy and began to love my hair because it was nappy.

There is nothing quite as versatile as nappy hair. One day it can be in twists, the next day it's in a gorgeous twist-out. Two days later, I can rock a wash-and-go. That night I can stretch it and wear a big afro the next day. If I get tired of that, I can brush it back into a puff. I could go on and on.

The moral of the story is that if your hair isn't what you'd expected it would be after the big chop, don't give up. Love it through the dry, rough scab hair stage, the "I want coils, but they aren't there" stage, and even the "This product isn't working!" stage. Be patient and you will find that you cannot beat the coily or coil-less tresses with which you've been blessed.

LV Burns, after having relaxed her hair for more than twenty years, cut off her relaxed hair in 2005 and has never looked back. LV's blog, *Natural-ness: A Journey Through the Lengths and Towards Healthy Living,* follows her transition from permed hair to natural hair. In showing new and future naturals her journey, she hopes to inspire and support those who have chosen to be their natural best. Through her comic strip, *Val and Nadine,* product reviews, and natural hair videos, she shows that the natural journey should be about learning to love, care for, and experiment with your natural hair.

Remember, when you make a commitment to natural hair, you don't make a commitment to the idea of natural hair or natural hair as a movement. You're making a commitment to your *specific* head of hair. So before you abandon your natural do because it wasn't everything you expected it to be, do yourself a favor and at least get to know your hair and spend time taking care of it so that you can deepen your commitment and fall in love with your natural do. Before you go running back to your relaxer, give due diligence to this new style. This is the time to become a product junkie and to experiment as much as you can. Use this new beginning to find out what both you and your hair like, and hopefully you'll be growing together for many years to come.

FINDING YOUR PERFECT TWA ROUTINE

Here's the funny thing about routines: in order to find the perfect one, you've got to do a lot of experimentation. For most of your life, having natural hair rather than getting it permed will save you money. But in the beginning, we actually suggest spending the money that used to go toward your hair appointments on new hair products. Yes, at the beginning of your natural hair journey, we suggest becoming a product junkie.

We kid! We kid! But we do seriously want to encourage you to experiment with several different products during this phase of your journey. A lot of women go into their natural hair

product junkie \ˈprä-(ˌ)dəkt ˈjəŋ-kē\

[noun]

Someone who buys excessive amounts of natural hair products. You can tell if someone you know is a product junkie just by observing her bathroom. If much of what you find underneath the bathroom sink is partially used bottles of products dating back to the year of her big chop, then you are probably dealing with a product junkie. If she refuses to learn how to cook, but you find more than three food-based oils (e.g., avocado oil, coconut oil, almond oil, olive oil) on top of her bathroom counter, then you are probably dealing with a product junkie. If she cannot find Morocco on a map but has an Internet site from which she orders a certain brand of Moroccan oil and a stash of the cheaper, impure version just in case she runs out of the good stuff, then you are probably dealing with a product junkie. If she lives in a trendy, gentrified neighborhood but can tell you where every beauty-supply shop that sells Fantasia IC gel is within a fifty-mile radius, then you are probably dealing with a product junkie.

journey with a preconceived agenda. A woman might want to use the exact same products that her cousin swears by, or she might decide that she will *only* use 100 percent natural products in her hair.

"I had a friend who was like, 'I don't put anything on my hair that I can't put in my mouth!'" says one curlfriend. "And I wanted to be like that, too. But my hair just didn't respond to the natural products the way it responded to the stuff with chemicals in it."

At the end of this book, you'll find an extensive product

guide. It's extensive because there are a lot of products out there that will work for your hair and a lot that won't. We don't recommend one product over another because, quite frankly, not every woman will be able to achieve a fierce twist-out with kitchen staples. Some of you will find that only certain products will achieve certain looks, and you'll have to experiment to find out what those products are.

That said, any TWA routine can basically be broken down into three categories: washing, styling, and maintenance.

WASHING YOUR TWA

Washing natural hair isn't like washing relaxed hair. Depending on hair length, it's either way easier or just a scooch harder. You have a few options for washing your hair:

1. You can shampoo once a week.
2. You can co-wash twice a week.
3. You can pre-poo with an oil or a conditioner, rinse that out, shampoo, and then condition once more.

Nikki's Instructions for Basic Hair Washing with Shampoo

STEP 1 Pick a shampoo with an active cleansing agent such as cocamidopropyl betaine. It's milder than sodium lauryl sulfate but is very effective at removing

pre-poo \(ˌ)prē-ˈpü\

[noun]

A pre-poo (also called pre-shampoo) is a treatment applied prior to shampooing that consists of oils and/or conditioners. It is usually performed to help the hair retain necessary moisture during the drying shampoo process. The cleansing process, while necessary, can be stressful on our delicate strands. Shampoo can strip the hair of vital oils and leave strands rough and tangled. Pre-poo treatments prevent the hair from absorbing too much water, which greatly reduces hygral fatigue (the expanding and contracting of hair as water enters and exits). These treatments also help maintain the structural integrity of your hair's cuticle and cortex. Finally, pre-pooing makes hair easier to detangle, which results in less breakage when it's combed. (See our product guide in the appendix for a list of pre-poos.)

excess oils and buildup. The excess oil needs to be cleansed away regularly for your scalp to stay healthy. Plus, leaving product residue on your hair will cause tangles and breakage. You have to cleanse thoroughly, but gently, and there are plenty of shampoos that can do that. (See our product guide in the appendix for shampoo options.)

STEP 2 Dilute the shampoo: Add a few tablespoons of shampoo to a large applicator bottle (which you can buy at a beauty-supply store such as Sally's). Mix in warm water for a 1:1 ratio, then shake vigorously. You want the mixture to be just a tad bit thicker than water but still very runny and easy to distribute throughout your scalp.

Benefits: More bang for your buck, helps to further stretch your favorite shampoo, efficiently targets the scalp, and is far less concentrated.

STEP 3 Thoroughly wet your hair, preferably in the shower, with warm water to help loosen up dirt.

STEP 4 Apply the shampoo mixture to your scalp with the applicator bottle.

STEP 5 Massage your scalp gently with your finger pads.

STEP 6 Rinse your hair thoroughly.

STEP 7 Follow up with an instant conditioner. (See our product guide in the appendix for ideas.)

STEP 8 Rinse your hair with cool water to seal and smooth the cuticles.

co-wash \kō-wäsh\

[verb]

Washing your hair with conditioner as opposed to shampoo. Many conditioners have enough cleansing properties to effectively clear away debris. This is a great way to retain moisture and allows for more frequent cleansing, as the conditioner doesn't strip your hair of its natural oils. You'll be left with soft, shiny, stronger tresses. However, it's important to note that if you're using silicone-laden and other less natural products, you'll have to use shampoo to cleanse. (See our product guide in the appendix for co-wash options.)

Co-washing

For co-washing, just follow the previous steps, replacing the shampoo with conditioner. There's no need to dilute the conditioner or to apply it with an applicator bottle, though.

DETANGLING
- -

No matter how short you big chop, within a year you'll be ready to start detangling your hair on wash days. If your hair is long enough to run a pick through, then it's long enough to detangle. See the three common detangling methods discussed in chapter 4 when you get to this point. We suggest trying each method at least once before deciding which one is best for you.

DEEP CONDITIONING
- -

At this stage, you should already be deep conditioning at every single wash session. Either beforehand, on dirty, dry hair, or on freshly cleansed and damp hair. If you deep condition regularly, you'll notice that your strands will be much less susceptible to breakage and split ends.

The best way to do a deep conditioning treatment is to divide your hair into sections and apply a generous amount of deep conditioner to your hair. Don a plastic cap for 15 to 30 minutes. Employing a gentle heat source will help the conditioner set in. (See Your Best Curlfriend Says on page 54 for details.) Finally, rinse out the deep conditioner with cool water.

Nikki's Supereasy Deep Conditioning Recipe

What you'll need:

¼ cup honey

¼ cup olive oil

Directions:

Mix the honey with the olive oil. Heat the mixture in a microwave until it melts and then apply it to your hair. Cover your head with a plastic cap for 15 to 30 minutes. To ramp up the moisturizing benefits, don a micro heat cap.

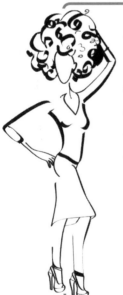

Your Best Curlfriend Says . . .

There are a few things you can do to provide your hair with the heat that it needs for a deep conditioning treatment to truly work. You can work out during the time it's setting, which is also good for hair growth, body, and mood. If you don't want to exercise, opt for gentle heat. Use a micro heat cap or wrap a warm, wet towel around your hair for moist heat. *Sitting under a bonnet dryer for extended times, even with a plastic cap on, can do more harm than good to your hair.* Gentle heat is always the way to go.

STYLING YOUR TWA

The Wash-and-Go

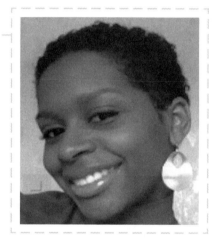

Superbusy and always on the move? The wash-and-go is the perfect style for you. All you have to do is wash your hair, put in some leave-in conditioner, followed by a cream or gel styler, then seal it with a little oil. For the best, frizz-free definition, allow your curls to dry without any manipulation. No touching!

Maintenance: Every morning spritz your hair with either a leave-in conditioner or a conditioner-water mixture and just go. Easy-peasy.

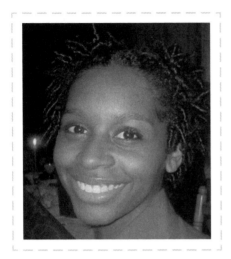

STEP 1 Wash and condition your hair.

STEP 2 Blot with a microfiber towel to remove excess water.

STEP 3 Apply a leave-in conditioner of your choice.

STEP 4 Using a comb or your fingers, divide your hair into four sections, two at the front and two at the back.

STEP 5 Start with the back, left section. Further divide that section into smaller square parts.

STEP 6 Apply the styler of your choice to your hair and distribute evenly.

STEP 7 Wrap your hair around the tail end of a rat

rat tail comb \rat tāl kōm\

[noun]

A favorite tool of curlfriends worldwide. A rat tail comb can be used to part hair, make curls, and smooth previously detangled hair prior to roller setting. A rat tail comb has a comb section with close teeth, and a much thinner "tail" made out of either metal or plastic. Many curlfriends prefer to use the metal tail for parting, especially if they are working with looser curls. But those with tighter curls might prefer the plastic tail, which gets the job done no matter what. However, both are so cheap that many curlfriends buy one of each.

tail comb. Twirl the comb slowly in a clockwise direction while pulling the comb out of the coil.

STEP 8 Repeat Step 7 until your entire head is complete.

If your length allows, you can use your fingers to style your hair in place of the rat tail comb.

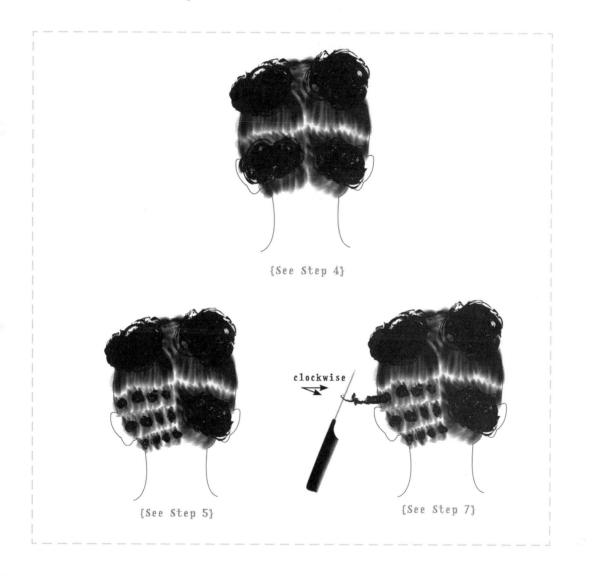

{See Step 4}

clockwise

{See Step 5}   {See Step 7}

A Message from Your Future Fro

By Alexandra Smith

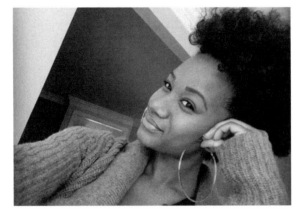

Is my hair growing or isn't it? That is the question. Most of us curly girls have gone through that "OMG, will I ever have something besides a TWA" phase. I personally have been there and know exactly how new naturals feel. It took my hair forever, and I took a lot of pictures to actually see that, yes, my hair was indeed growing.

For those of you who choose to big chop versus transition for a year or more, I would suggest that you take a lot of pictures to document your progress. Also, when you are feeling discouraged about your new head of hair, check out natural hair videos on YouTube for a pick-me-up. This journey is a beautiful one but may not be as easy for some as it is for others, and that's okay!

Honestly, I think the struggles we go through as naturals are what make our journey so meaningful. The trial and error of it all can be extremely beneficial in the long run. I've been natural for two years, and this is my third (and final) attempt to embrace my mane.

I think being natural worked this time around because I was not only patient and confident in my choice, but I was also satisfied with my hair. When I say satisfied, I mean I learned to love every inch of my kinky coils. No one could convince me that what I had sprouting from my scalp wasn't beautiful. We all might face the mini-bush blues during our journey. Heck, some of us may even have big-bush blues days, but after all is said and done, those bush blues are beautiful.

The natural hair community is full of knowledge just for us, and fellow curly girls are more than willing to help shed light on anything and everything relating to curly hair and confidence. This hair choice should be a fun learning experience, not a task! To all of you newbie naturals, I wish you the best of luck and many years of happy hair growing.

Alexandra Smith is a young single mother of one, a full-time media journalism student, and a business owner. She shares her curly girl experience and other kinky hair goodness on *The Good Hair Blog*. Her overall goal for blogging is to bring the natural hair community together, men included, by spreading knowledge, inspiration, and love about our diverse heads of hair.

Flat Twists in Front, Leave the Rest Out

STEP 1 Wash and condition your hair.

STEP 2 Blot your hair with a microfiber towel to remove excess water.

STEP 3 Add a leave-in conditioner throughout your hair.

STEP 4 Part your hair horizontally, with the part running over the top of your head from ear to ear, and secure the back half with an ouchless hair band.

STEP 5 Make a vertical part (about an inch up from your ear) from your hairline back to the original part.

STEP 6 Secure the rest of the hair in the front section out of the way with an ouchless band.

STEP 7 With a bit of styler on your fingertips, take some of the loose section nearest to your face and split *that* portion into two pieces.

STEP 8 Twist those two pieces of hair around each other, gently incorporating hair from the loose section into the twist as you work back toward the ear-to-ear part. Don't twist too tight!

STEP 9 Some textures will hold the twist with no assistance, but if you must, use a bobby pin or clip to secure the twist in place.

STEP 10 Repeat Steps 7 to 9 until you're done.

STEP 11 Add leave-in conditioner to the back, a bit of styler, and you're done!

Optional: If you want more curl definition in the back, take a few more minutes to add some styler to your fingertips and lightly tweak as many curls as you can.

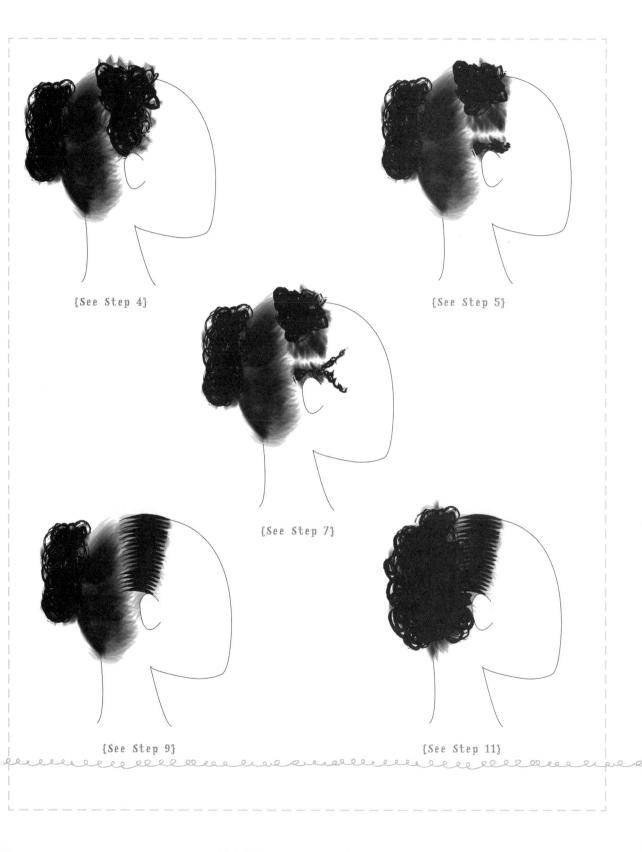

{See Step 4}

{See Step 5}

{See Step 7}

{See Step 9}

{See Step 11}

Pin Back the Front, Leave the Rest Out

This is as simple as it sounds. Play around with different parts—side, middle, diagonal—and pin and tuck as you see fit. Leave the back of your hair out for a cute style!

Accessorize with a Headband or a Scarf

Head to Target, Forever 21, or a similar discount store, and go on a scarf spree! You'll be surprised at the cheap finds and how something so simple can do so much for your style!

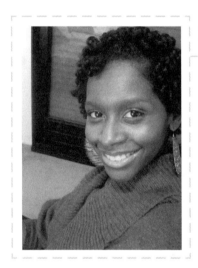

Bantu Knots

STEP 1 On dry, damp, or wet hair, create two-strand twists throughout your entire head. (Simply take two strands of hair and twist them around each other from root to tip.)

STEP 2 Twirl each twist until it buckles on itself and wrap the length around the bottom of the loop, then tuck the end into the "o" loop. Literally tie the twist into a knot.

STEP 3 Allow time to set and then release the knots to reveal an s-wave texture!

Enjoy this time with your TWA. Right now, styling is short and sweet, but later on you'll need to invest a little more time. Even if you're pining for longer hair, believe us, you'll eventually come to miss the newborn years.

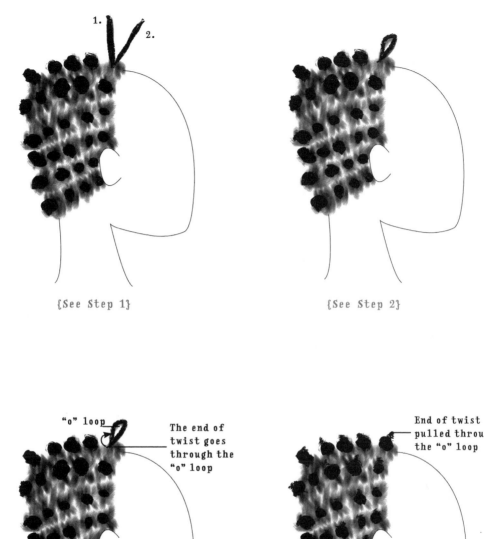

1.
2.

{See Step 1}

{See Step 2}

"o" loop

The end of twist goes through the "o" loop

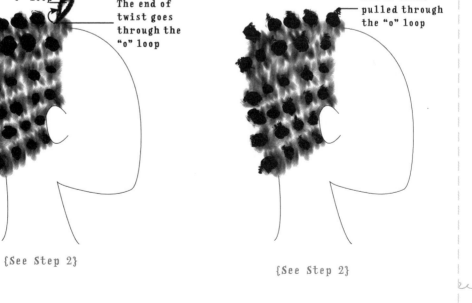

End of twist pulled through the "o" loop

{See Step 2}

{See Step 2}

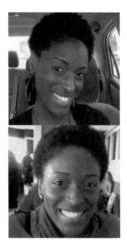

Right now, I love the wash-and-go with my TWA. I can't wait until it gets longer so I can have a puff! Being natural gave me a whole new excuse to reinvent myself and my style. I'm always out looking for a new bow to accent my TWA. This process has been exciting for me, and it's only just beginning.

—REANELL FREDERICK

TIPS FOR TERRIFIC TWAs

* Give your new or proposed routine at least three weeks so that you can do a proper assessment of whether it's right for you.
* Try one product at a time so you know what works.
* Eliminate one product at a time from a failed routine so that you can easily identify exactly what isn't working.
* It's best to apply oil to your hair when it's wet. This will help your hair hold in the moisture that's already on the hair shaft.
* Use water. Water is by far the best moisturizer known to man. In between a styling session, simply dampen the hair, then seal in the moisture with a light oil such as jojoba or grape seed oil. Use a spray bottle for easy application.
* Refresh a matted TWA by spritzing it with an oil mixture (your favorite hair care ingredients together in one bottle, which you can spray on your hair whenever it's needed). An oil mixture can consist of your favorite oils, or it can be a blend of vegetable glycerin and your favorite oils, or you can try aloe vera juice or conditioner plus a little water and your favorite oil.
* Remember, as comedian Wanda Sykes told Nikki in reference to her own hair, "It's a damn science lab," and she wasn't joking!

TWA WEARERS SOUND OFF!

I had transitioned for six months once before and went to do the big chop and got nervous and got a relaxer and then regretted it, so I knew I was ready to make the switch to natural hair. It was definitely freeing and liberating! I had an awesome time with my cousins finding big earrings and other fun accessories to complement my new style, and I'm loving the experience. God has been doing some major internal work on me, and I felt like this was the outward expression of the change and letting go of the old me. —Nikevia Latrice Bowie

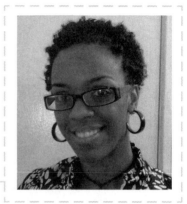

My first reaction to seeing my finished big chop consisted of several stages. First, I thought, I can't believe I just did this. *Then I thought,* I love this. *Next I thought,* This is going to take some getting used to. *And finally I thought,* I'm sooo glad I did this. *I did the big chop in a professional salon, so I decided to have my hair cut into a shape (longer on the top and shorter at the back and sides) and to have it colored red. So my hairstyle itself needs no accessories and, in fact, is my best accessory. Today, I'm enjoying watching my hair's evolution. It's still fly. Going natural was one of the best decisions I've made, and I'm looking forward to experimenting with different styles, shapes, and colors at every length.* —Briaan L. Barron

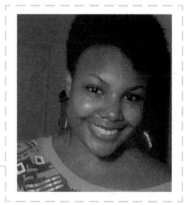

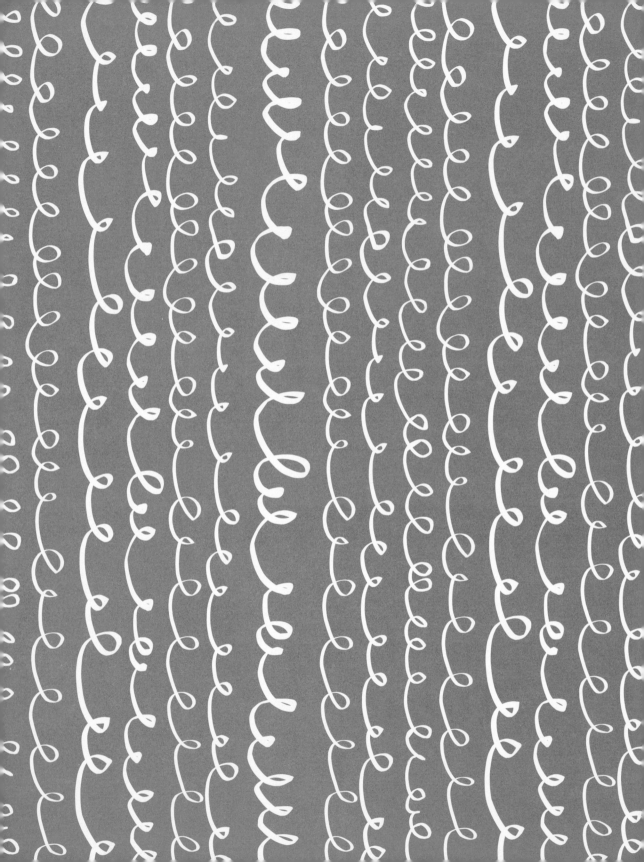

CHAPTER THREE

The Terrible Twos

Standing By Your Hair— Even When It's Acting a Fool

When we talk about the terrible twos in terms of hair, we're not talking about the age of your natural, so much as a particular phase that most of us will hit after we leave the TWA stage behind—a stage that might involve some crying and the occasional tantrum.

At this point in your natural hair journey, you should have a few things going for you:

* Depending on the length of your hair after your big chop, you've found at least one or two styles that you can do easily and efficiently.
* Your family and/or friends are no longer giving you a hard time about your hair length.
* Your significant other has accepted your hair or the relationship has ended.
* You've found products that your hair loves and that fit within your budget.
* No matter how you felt at the time of your big chop, you've become accustomed to rocking natural hair now.

But just as everything is going smoothly on your natural hair journey, suddenly your locks decide to get a mind of their own. You know your hair has hit the terrible twos, when one or more of the following happens:

1. YOUR HAIR BECOMES A TOTAL BRAT. Hairstyles that used to look good just don't anymore. And you start having a lot of bad hair days. Your hair starts arbitrarily rejecting the products it used to love, and sometimes it sticks its tongue out at you when you're trying to put in your tried-and-true, go-to styles. Much like the mom who doesn't know whether her toddler will pitch a fit in the grocery store or sit quietly in the cart like a perfect angel, you have no idea going into a styling session if your hair will turn out the way you want it to. Your wash-and-go becomes a wash-and-oh-no because you're too fearful

to attempt one, since you no longer know what you're going to get.

2. YOU'RE BORED, BORED, *BORED*! Your best styles just aren't popping the way they used to. And you're starting to feel the love you used to have for your natural hair wane.

3. YOU'RE LOSING MOTIVATION. Getting to know your natural hair used to be a fun experiment, but now you find that you're having more problems with itchy scalp, because you keep putting off washing your hair. Your hair has become a total chore—one you don't feel like doing.

4. YOU'RE NO LONGER GETTING COMPLIMENTS. Everyone you know, including your boo (aka your main compliment source) has become used to your hair, and the honeymoon is definitely over. It's kind of like how our little ones' pictures get fewer and fewer "likes" on Facebook the older the kids get.

5. YOU'VE SOMEHOW AMASSED A DISTURBINGLY LARGE COLLECTION OF HATS. And it would really upset you if you lost your favorite one. We mean really upset you in the same way it would upset a toddler if she lost her security blanket.

Moms often lament having to deal with the stuff that wasn't in the "having kids brochure," such as dealing with grown-up-level poop, the sometimes mind-numbing boredom, public temper tantrums, and failed potty-training sessions (which brings us right back to the grown-up poop). It's eerie how much your natural hair's awkward phase can feel

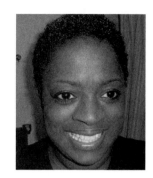

When I began this journey, my goal was healthy hair; I never wanted length. I just made sixteen months from my first big chop, and I can't say that I will allow it to get as long this time. As long as my hair is healthy, I am happy.

—GAYE GLASSPIE

exactly like trying to manage a child in the throes of her terrible twos.

This stage is short (usually you're out of it within a year), but it's powerful because this is when a lot of naturals get frustrated and go back to relaxers or big chop once again and start all over. There's nothing wrong with going back to a TWA if you find that you really are more comfortable at that stage. Curlfriend Gaye Glasspie told us that her hair, which she's nicknamed Sasha, grew too fast, and she ended up getting it cut again sixteen months after her big chop.

Another curlfriend we know considers getting her locks shorn every three months a marriage saver. "My husband and I both agree that I'm much saner when I keep my hair short." Indeed, if you find yourself becoming obsessed with hair maintenance in ways that affect your relationships or self-worth, wearing it short might be the way to go.

TWAs can also be a great look and a practical move for busy moms and career women alike. Long hair is great, but keep in mind that short and sweet just may be the best hair fit for your lifestyle.

However, also remember that the terrible twos stage is exactly that—a stage. Most of our curlfriends who have cut their hair during this awkward phase have later expressed regret about doing so. They wish they had been more patient, and they vow to do better the next time around.

Remember, if your main goal is length, you can't and won't achieve it without being patient. Like the stay-at-home mom who will one day send her fully potty-trained child off to kindergarten, you just have to manage the terrible twos as best you can if you want to make it to the magical five-year mark (which we'll talk about in chapter 4).

And this is where we come in. In this chapter, you'll find hairstyles, tips, and lots of commiseration. You're not alone. We're here to help you through the terrible twos.

GIVE YOUR HAIR A TIME-OUT

First, if you're getting close to reaching for the creamy crack, *stop*. We ask that you give it at least a month before you decide to relax your hair again. Much the same way that mommies sometimes need a break from their toddlers, it might behoove you to take some time off from your hair. Here are a few ideas about how to do this.

*   DO THIRTY DAYS OF PROTECTIVE STYLES. Putting your hair in a protective style means you don't have to bother with it. No need to do a twist-*out* when you can just wear twists for a little while. Protective styles are a great way to give your hair a break from styling.
*   PUT YOUR HAIR IN BRAIDS. Braids are versatile and easy to take care of. And if you don't feel like using synthetic hair, no problem. You can get your own hair cornrowed in any style, from an elegant bun that's perfect for work to a funky mohawk that you can wear until you're ready to deal with your hair again.
*   WEAR A WIG. Wigs are not just for your grandma anymore, and they come in all sorts of natural

options these days. One curlfriend says, "It's my go-to whenever I'm frustrated with my hair, or whenever I want to hide it for a boost in undisturbed growth!"

* GET A WEAVE. Yes, girl, we said it. (We told you that we weren't your typical natural hair bible.) Quiet as it's kept, weaves come in natural versions as well. In fact, some of our favorite curlebrities secretly sport them. Weaves serve the double purpose of giving you the length you desire and a break from styling.

* MAKE AN APPOINTMENT AT A NATURAL HAIR SALON. If just the thought of spending another minute tending to your natural hair is setting your teeth on edge, go to the CurlyNikki forums and find a great natural hairstylist in your area. A fabulous professional protective style, such as braids, might be just the thing to get you past your hair funk.

After you take your month off from styling your hair, consider doing the following to prevent a relapse back into hair boredom.

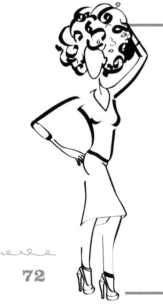

Your Best Curlfriend Says . . .

Washing and deep conditioning your hair the night before your scheduled hair appointment will save you both time and money. Be sure to let your stylist know ahead of time that you'll be coming in only to get your hair braided. Also, if possible, book the first appointment of the morning. That way you won't have to sit around waiting for your stylist to finish up with the person who came in before you.

FIND YOUR PERFECT LAZY HAIR ROUTINE. You don't have to look like you just stepped out of an *Essence* photo shoot every day. Find a style that takes the least amount of work and go with that until you hit a nonawkward length.

DO A TEN-STYLE HAIR CHALLENGE. Like most naturals, you probably have a folder on your computer full of pictures and/or how-to videos for styles you'd like to try. Try them now! If you don't have a "someday" folder, even better. Go to YouTube and search for "natural hair updos" or "natural hair styles." Pick the top ten styles you'd like to try and spend the next two months running through them all. This is a great way to pass the time while waiting for your hair to grow, and it just might snap you out of your hair boredom.

SPEND MORE TIME ON YOUR HAIR. This solution seems counterintuitive—you're sick of your fro right now and you're a few bad hair days away from cutting it off altogether. But just as a romantic weekend often rejuvenates couples on the brink of divorce, spending even more time on your hair than you normally do might make you love it more. Take out your calendar and schedule a monthly date night with your hair for the next six months. Decide ahead of time what you and your hair are going to "do" that night. For example, our vision of a perfect hair-date night would involve pampering ourselves with a homemade deep conditioning treatment, then listening to a favorite CD while we style our hair, with a glass of wine and a box of chocolates nearby. You'll be surprised by how much you'll come to treasure these special times spent pampering your hair.

NATURAL VS. COMMERCIAL

One of the big decisions that every natural will have to make for herself is how natural she wants to be. For some women, the natural hair journey is very spiritual and is part of a lifestyle overhaul that might also include adopting a vegetarian or vegan diet and attaining better mental health. If your original reasons for going natural were spiritual, at the terrible twos point you might want to take on the challenge of going all-natural. There are many all-natural options in the appendix. Here are a few pros and cons of living an all-natural lifestyle.

Pros

* Fewer issues with product buildup.
* No need for frequent washes or harsh sulfate-laden shampoos.
* Can cheaply and efficiently make products using ingredients from your kitchen.
* Fewer health consequences. (Research shows that chemicals from hair products can seep into the

bloodstream. If there are no toxins or carcinogens in your products, you don't have to worry about this.)

Cons

* Hair might be less manageable and more difficult to detangle (chemical labs have created some pretty awesome formulas to melt away tangles).
* No running to the nearest store to pick up your hair supplies (all-natural products may be harder to find).
* Natural products have a shorter shelf life. You'll have to keep them refrigerated or risk mold. (We hate applying cold hair products, but we hate moldy ones even more.)
* Some natural hair products can get pricey (twenty bucks for four ounces of argan oil, etc.).

If you're already only using all-natural products, you might want to consider embracing the nonorganic products that naturals used back in the day. Products like Blue Magic grease, Luster's Pink Original Hair Lotion, and old-school oil sheens tend to be cheaper than their all-natural counterparts, and some of our curlfriends have reported getting better results with these oldies but goodies than with the more expensive all-natural products.

At the beginning of this latest incarnation of the natural hair movement, the need to keep everything that went on your hair *pure* was stressed. But as the movement grows in size and scope, many curlfriends are embracing natural products while holding on to a few of the staple products they grew up with.

Why I Keep It *All*-Natural

By Sherrell Dorsey

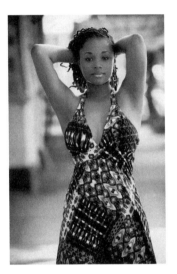

Making the decision to use organic and natural hair products just made sense for me. After all, I ditched the creamy crack, tossed the chemical damage aside, and liberated my hair to become healthy and free. Why would I ruin my hair's rehab program by continuing to use products that are laden with potentially carcinogenic chemicals? It just doesn't make sense. Especially when there are more than enough products on the market, not to mention Grandma's old kitchen recipes, that are free from harsh ingredients and keep my natural hair, well, natural.

Years ago I could buy into the excuse that going green and organic was too expensive, but now I refuse to accept the typical defense that most people use simply because they don't want to shell out a few extra dollars. I still Google recipes for dry scalp and hair issues and get lots of information from blogs and YouTube videos to continue learning about how I can take care of my hair. It's not rocket science; it's just smart. Plus, I *never* have to pop into the beauty-supply store and waste my money on some mystery grease experiment flown in from who-knows-where and sold to me from vendors who can't even educate me on the product.

My natural and organic hair products last longer and work

better simply because they contain fewer fillers and less water, so I'm actually getting a more concentrated mix of power ingredients feeding my hair (not to mention my money's worth). Before there was a Pantene Pro-V, a JAM, or Luster's Pink Lotion, there was shea butter, olive oil, jojoba oil, and argan oil, and guess what? They all worked.

Why I'm Just *Sorta* Natural

By GG Renee Hill

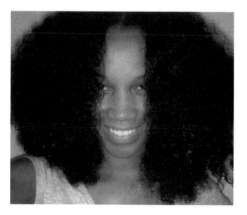

The transition from relaxed to natural hair is an incredibly eye-opening experience, particularly when it comes to how to care for your hair. Prior to my transition, I never thought of my natural hair as curly. Matter of fact, I never thought much about my hair texture at all. Gradually, I learned that my hair was curly in some places, wavy here and there, and extremely thick and indefinable on the top. My hair's multiple personalities mystified me, and I found myself looking for a holy grail product that would make all the various textures cooperate. Eventually, I had to take a step back and consider whether I should even be using the same products on my natural hair that I had always used on my relaxed hair.

This was tough for me. I had to reevaluate everything I knew about caring for my previously straight hair. As I began to research natural hair, I was overwhelmed with information about what ingredients curly girls should avoid and why. With no particular rhyme or reason, I just began trying things. I cut out sulfates, heavy silicones, and mineral oil altogether. I experimented with natural and homemade products, as I learned that they would cause less buildup on my hair and moisturize it more effectively. I observed positive changes right away, and over time I amassed an arsenal of new staples.

This discovery process came full circle one day when I ran out of my favorite sealer and had to use some hair grease that was collecting dust in the back of my closet. The next day, I unraveled one of the most defined twist-outs I have ever had, and it lasted for days. Just like that, I reopened my mind to the option of strategically using products with less desirable ingredients. I love having these additional options now that I have learned how to manage them. With moderate use and a good clarifying shampoo, I can use products with "bad" ingredients to accomplish certain styling goals. Meanwhile, my hair continues to benefit from the nutrients in natural products and the effects of deep conditioning, layering moisture, and sealing.

Ultimately, we all have priorities that affect how we care for our hair, and they are bound to change over time. The philosophy that has worked for me is to keep an open mind and an active sense of curiosity. There's nothing like the sense of awareness that comes from identifying your own unique needs and the solutions that work best for you.

It's up to every natural to decide for herself whether to use all-natural hair products, whatever other products work on her hair, or a mixture of both.

THE FIVE ORGANIC PRODUCTS *ALL* CURLFRIENDS SHOULD HAVE IN THEIR COLLECTION

1. SHEA BUTTER. It restores moisture and softness to thirsty tresses from the root to the tip. It's even beneficial for dry, itchy scalp. Shea butter has also been known to tame and "clump" curls, as well as reduce frizz—so it's a natural pomade! It also will protect your hair from damage due to the weather, dryness, and brittleness.

2. ALOE VERA. This magical extract protects your hair from heat damage. It has a low pH (just like our hair), and it smooths the hair cuticle and defines curls like no other! It enhances shine and can be beneficial in the detangling process. It is light and won't weigh down your curls. Aloe vera also provides a light hold without the "crunch" factor of other products.

3. JOJOBA EXTRACT. It heals dry and damaged hair while restoring shine and softness. Like shea butter, it clumps curls and helps to reduce frizz. Jojoba most closely resembles the body's natural oil and is okay to use from your hair's root to the tip. Like shea

butter, it will protect your hair from wind damage, brittleness, and dryness. It doesn't necessarily moisturize the hair as much as it nourishes your tresses, so be sure to use a moisturizing water-based conditioner, moisturizer, or leave-in conditioner under this oil. It will do an excellent job at sealing in the benefits of whatever moisturizer you use.

4. EXTRA VIRGIN OLIVE OIL is an emollient that seals and softens the hair. You can add it to a conditioner for extra slip (extra moisturizing), or use it as a quick pre-shampoo or a deep conditioner.

5. HONEY is a light humectant that also has antibacterial properties. You can add it to your conditioner and deep conditioner for extra slip and a moisture punch. It's also great as a final rinse, and some curlfriends even use a tiny bit, emulsified in water, as a leave-in! Shiny, shiny, defined hair!

GETTING YOUR HAIR TO HANG

One of the biggest frustrations with awkward length is getting the hair to "hang"—that is, getting it to face downward as opposed to facing upward and outward. When your hair is at its most awkward length, the grass often appears greener on the longer side. But trust us when we say that you'll eventually come to miss having hair that can stand up without a ton of manipulation and heavy product use on your part. But until that day comes, here are a few tips to get more hang time from your fro.

1. FLAT-TWIST OR PIN YOUR ROOTS. Often when our curlfriends two-strand-twist their hair, the roots unravel, leaving them with results that are half-poofy and undefined. To achieve even definition from root to tip, begin each twist by flat-twisting the hair to your scalp. On lazy days, do a simple two-strand twist, but use a bobby pin to pin the root to your scalp. Both techniques allow for better definition, with the unexpected side effect of better hang time! Using this technique on wet or damp hair reduces shrinkage as well.

2. USE A SATIN OR SILK SCARF TO SET YOUR HAIR. In line with the first tip, once your hair is twisted, reach for your satin or silk scarf and tie down your crown (like a pirate). This will help to set your hair in the downward position. Do this whether you've twisted wet or dry hair, and if you sleep in your twists, tie on the scarf prior to donning your satin cap.

3. **ROLL THE ENDS.** Simply twist your hair and set the last two inches or so on a roller. It gives supercute definition, and on wet hair, it adds weight to each twist, which reduces shrinkage. This tip used in conjunction with the first two tips should be your best bet.

4. **TENSION DRY BEFORE TWISTING.** To get the most hang time on hair that is styled dry, retwist an old twist-out or blow out your freshly cleansed, moisturized hair. If you choose to blow-dry your hair, use the tension method in which you simply stretch your hair with one hand and, holding the blow-dryer in a downward motion, blast your roots with warm (not hot) heat. It's less manipulation than your typical blow out, and it gently straightens your roots, which will result in some downward hanging.

5. **RETHINK THE PRODUCTS YOU USE.** Heavier products weigh down hair. Hair that is weighed down is less likely to rise. If it's hang time you seek, opt for a moisturizing leave-in *plus* a styler, such as a gel, butter, or pomade, and be liberal with your application! This tip works best on wet-set twist-outs.

Remember, some hair textures don't really allow for hang time, no matter what you try. We've also found that with length comes weight, and that added weight helps hair to hang where it didn't before. It's important to remember to work with what you've got! Don't fight your hair. If it wants to reach toward the sky, you'll be a lot less frustrated if you embrace that fact and work with it, not against it!

EVEN MORE TIPS FOR DEALING WITH AWKWARD HAIR LENGTHS

* Do twist-outs, braid-outs, or roller sets to show off your hard-earned length.

    I reach for the bottle of olive oil, get some coconut oil and mix in some sweet almond oil with my conditioner, and let my curls soak it up. I found that a good deep conditioning treatment helps to get my hair back in shape. —*Namun*

* Enjoy the volume now, because the longer your hair gets, the harder it'll be to get height at the crown. So rock it tall. Block movie theater screens and other folks' view behind you at the concert.

    When my hair pisses me off and doesn't act right, I load it with curl friendly gel and put it into a pouf. Within a few days, after it's tired of being in hair jail, I will do a shampoo, condition, deep condition, and then see where it's at. Most times, it's back to normal. —*L. Michelle*

* Get a supercute shape-up. It'll make a world of difference and help you get past this stage in a fashionable way! A lot of curlfriends experience patches of hair that grow faster than others. If you've developed a shag (not cute), don't hang on to it for the sake of having longer hair. The perfect shape can be key for curly styles.

* Keep a journal. Take pictures of your hair and keep a record of styles that worked and what product combos

yielded the best results. Although it seems that your growth has stalled, you'll be surprised at how much your hair has grown when you look back at the pictures.

What I do is try something new: It could be a style I used to wear years ago and haven't worn in a while. I go to YouTube to see what the girls are doing with their hair. I Google "natural hair styles" to see what comes up. I try to do something that is new at that time in my life. And if all else fails, I pay a professional to help me come up with something that is all new and all-natural."

—Jeanette

* Accessorize. Get new earrings and headbands; try a braided headband, hair flowers, and so on.

When I start to get irritated with my hair, I plan a "Me Day." I pamper myself with a long hair-washing session and deep condition. I do my own pedicure and manicure and then browse the blogs or watch TV while looking for new styles to try.

—Neem

* Try henna! (See chapter 4 for more information.)

If none of these tricks make you fall back in love with being natural, this is a good time to reassess whether it's what you really want. There's nothing wrong with moving back to your hometown after living in the big city. And there's nothing wrong with going back to relaxers if you're no longer deriving any happiness from being natural. We joke about the creamy crack, but this chapter isn't meant to make you feel guilty for going back to it. It's meant to help you make the best decision about what your next hair step should be. Don't cut or relax your hair in the midst of frustration. Deal with the frustration first, then make your decision. And if you *do* end up deciding to stand by your natural hair, then twist-outs, braid-outs, bantu knot-outs, and roller sets are a few of our favorite styles for awkward lengths. You can also try the following styles.

The Perfect Puff

STEP 1 Start with a fresh twist-out or a dry wash-and-go.

STEP 2 Pull the hair back using a Goody headband (wrapped twice) to create a massive puff or with a smaller Goody Ouchless band or hair tie to create a smaller version.

STEP 3 To smooth the edges, rub a pea-size amount of shea butter (or castor oil or grease) between your palms and apply it in a smoothing motion to your hairline. Then tie on a silk scarf for 30 minutes. This will help your edges lie down and look neat—the *perfect* puff.

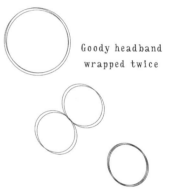

Goody headband
wrapped twice

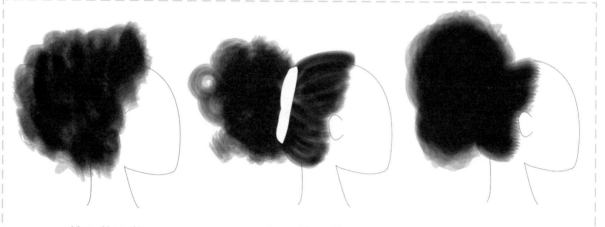

{See Step 1}   {See Step 2}   {See Step 3}

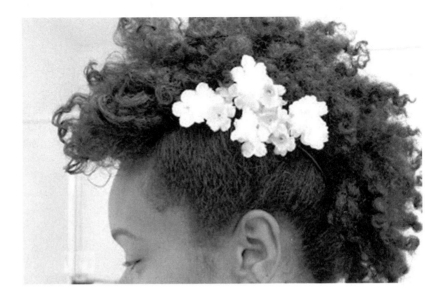

A Fierce Frohawk

Instructions provided by Alexandra Smith from The Good Hair Blog

What you'll need:

    Your favorite leave-in conditioner or refresher

    Styler: a hair gel, pomade, or butter-based moisturizer

    Spray bottle with water

    Shea butter

    Hooded dryer or micro heat cap

    Pick

    4 to 6 Goody side combs

    Bobby pins

STEP 1 Apply leave-in conditioner and styler to dry hair. (This is a great style for two- to five-day-old hair.)

STEP 2 Twist your hair. Do not bother with formal sections. Spritz each batch of hair with water before twisting. Put in ten to fifteen twists. After you finish each twist, seal the ends with shea butter.

STEP 3 Dry your hair for 15 minutes. Do not take the twists out while damp or your hair might come out frizzy.

STEP 4 Take the twists down. Separate each twist carefully, and then separate again so that you get four sections per twist.

STEP 5 Stretch your twists. Use a pick to stretch your roots upward for extra volume.

STEP 6 Make your frohawk. Simply pin the sides to your liking with the Goody combs and bobby pins. Frohawks are a very intuitive style, so don't be afraid to take the frohawk down and do it again until it looks just the way you want it to.

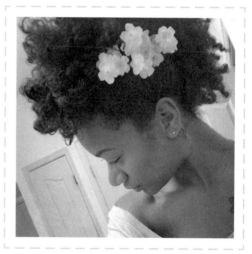

STEP 7 Add a fun hair accessory down the side. Flowers like the ones pictured are perfect. But play around with it. Hair accessories will give your frohawk that extra oomph!

Dry Twist-Out and Curl

Instructions provided by Savvy Brown from the blog Savvy Brown

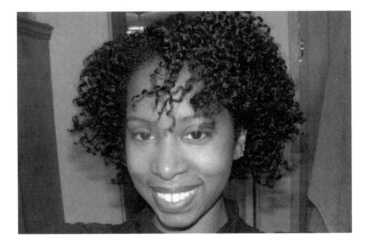

What you'll need:

Daily leave-in conditioner in spray form (you can
make your own: 1 part conditioner, 1 part water,
1 part oil; optional: a drop or two of your favorite
essential oil such as peppermint or jasmine)

Clips, pins, or ties for sectioning

Moisturizer (either a creamy leave-in conditioner or
butter or pudding)

Hair oil (Savvy loves castor oil for this style)

Holding spray (Savvy suggests Jane Carter Solution
Natural Hold Locking Spray)

Curlers

Optional: A rat tail comb for parting hair (your fingers
will work too)

STEP 1 Spritz your hair with conditioner, gently pulling the curls as you spritz to loosen them up.

STEP 2 To section the hair, make a part around the back of your head from earlobe to earlobe with your hands or a rat tail comb. Pin, clip, or tie the top section out of the way. Part the back into three sections, and clip two of those sections back.

STEP 3 Take a dab of moisturizer and run it through the unclipped section with your fingers (no combing or brushing!).

STEP 4 Separate the section you're working with into two smaller sections and twist each section as tight as you can all the way down to the ends.

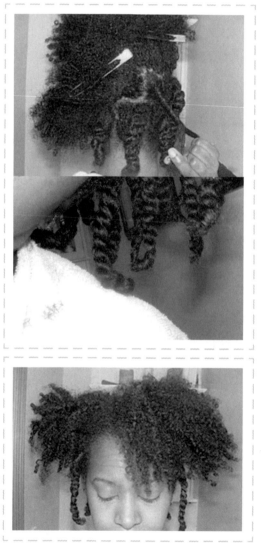

About a half inch from the end of the twist, seal your ends by dipping your fingers in whatever oil you've chosen. Finish twisting, then twirl the end on your finger to make sure it's covered in oil and to get nicely defined, unfrizzy curls.

You should have two separate twists when you're finished with the section. It's okay if they loosen a bit, but if a twist completely unravels, that means it's too big.

STEP 5 Repeat Steps 3 and 4 with the other section of hair. When you finish, the top part of your hair should umbrella above your twists.

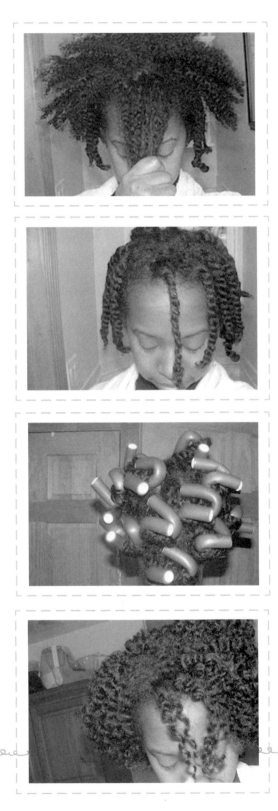

STEP 6 Make your part, either in the middle, to the left, or to the right, as Savvy has.

STEP 7 Clip or braid the bangs out of the way and to the side. You'll deal with this hair last.

STEP 8 Continue twisting your hair. Repeat Steps 3 and 4 on the top section in a circle until you come to the bangs you sectioned off.

STEP 9 Twist your bangs according to how you want them to lie. If you want a "stacked" look that falls in your face, make three or four smaller twists along the bang part line.

STEP 10 Spray each twist with holding spray and roll it up. Choose the size of the curler according to your preference and hair length. Keep in mind that the twists will need to sit for 5 hours at a minimum. So either choose a curler you're comfortable sleeping in or plan your day accordingly.

STEP 11 Unroll your twists.

STEP 12 Rub hair oil onto your hands and gently take down each twist. Pull each twist taut from the end of the hair and turn it in the opposite direction. Then use your fingers to separate the twists.

STEP 13 After all of the twists have been taken down, fluff your hair with your hands from the roots only. Then shake your head vigorously and turn your head upside down to fluff your hair some more. Work on the bangs last, using bobby pins to style it if the hair doesn't lie down the way you want.

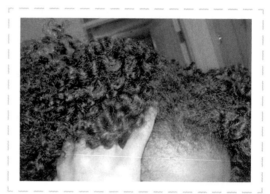

TERRIBLE TWOS SOUND OFF!

I am about six months shy of my two-year anniversary, and me and Ms. K (my hair) are not the best of friends at this moment. It seems like I just got out of the really awkward TWA phase where I felt I had to wear earrings just to be cute. I enjoyed my puff style for some time, then everything went haywire when my hair stopped responding to my holy grail products. So now, not only am I dealing with learning how to adjust to the length, but my products don't work! So not cool! In my picture I am rocking bantu knot-outs, a style that my hair loves at the moment.

—Shan'Terika Remo

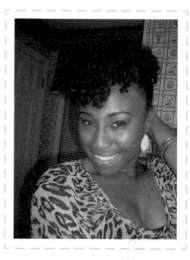

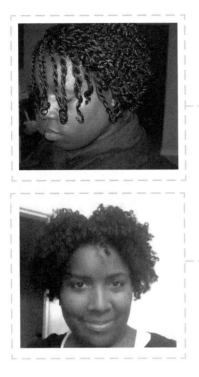

I have threatened my poor hair at least three times this week that I was going to do the big chop again! I have only not cut my hair because of protective updos and twists.

—Fern Illidge

I'm just short of the eighteen-month mark. I'm patiently waiting to move on from "standing up" to "hanging." I wear a lot of twist-outs, which are great because I like to pin my twists back or pull them back. I also wear a puff at least once a week. I like this stage because it forces you to try new things.

—Chantel Nattiel

CHAPTER FOUR

The Golden Years

It's Your Anniversary!

You know how excited children get when they "finally" make it to kindergarten? Well, that's nothing compared with the thrill of making it to the five-year mark as a natural. This is a golden time for most naturals that comes with greater hair confidence and access to even more hairstyles.

For the most part I love being natural because, for me, it means total acceptance of myself. This is me in totality. What you see is what you get. No more making myself or my hair conform to someone else's standards. Much like my style of dress, my hairstyles are versatile. I may

93

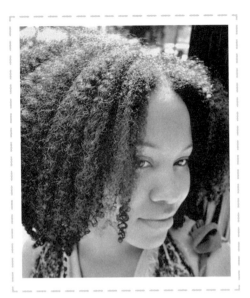

wear twists Monday through Friday, and a twist-out Saturday and Sunday. The next Monday I might decide to blow-dry and flat-iron and rock a sleek straight look. I love the fact that I don't have to keep up with when I had my last touch-up, take cover when it rains, roll my hair when I want some texture, be chemically bound to only straight hairstyles, blaze my scalp every six to eight weeks with sodium hydroxide, or wrap or roller set my hair after cleansing. Now, I have the freedom to do or not do whatever I want. Although I like trying new things, I'm no longer a product junkie. I'm happy to say that with time I've found my rhythm.
—Ebony Clark

At this point, your natural feels like a part of you. You're no longer frustrated with it, and going back to a relaxer or cutting off all your hair again is no longer a constant temptation. In short, by the five-year mark, you should be totally head over heels in love with your hair.

If you're not at the five-year mark yet, don't worry. Use this chapter for inspiration. When you consider giving up on your natural during its terrible twos—which a lot of us do—reread this chapter and recommit. If you can make it to the five-year mark, we can almost guarantee you'll be happy that you did.

Although this chapter is titled "The Golden Years," this section of the book, more than any other, is really meant for naturals at all stages. Here we'll cover a mishmash of tips, ideas, and issues that can pop up at any stage of your journey, such as figuring out how to detangle your hair, giving yourself hair trims, what to do with your hair while on vacation, and how to combat hair ennui. Our goal with this chapter is to give you the information and tools to have fabulous hair all the time. So if you read any chapter in this book, make sure to read this one.

DETANGLING

There are three common detangling methods. We recommend trying each method at least once and then trying them again every year or so just to make sure you're using the method your hair likes best.

Sink/Mirror Detangling

* Apply an oil (olive, coconut, argan, etc.) to soften, lubricate, and add slip (see the definition below). Some curlfriends dampen their hair with water first.
* Separate the hair into four to eight sections for easier handling.

slippage \sli-pij\

[noun]

How slippery a product is (usually a conditioner or a detangler). The more "slip" a product has, the more effectively it will coat the hair to aid in detangling.

* Choose a section and detangle gently with your fingers, working your way up from the ends to the roots, removing knots, tangles, and shedded hair.

   Optional: Comb through with a wide tooth comb or a paddle brush to be sure all shedded hairs have been removed.
* Twist this section and move on to the next. Repeat all over your head.
* Once in the shower, you can (1) shampoo and condition with the hair still in the twists/sections; (2) take down all of the twists, being careful not to retangle during the wash and condition process; or (3) take the twists down one section at time, shampoo, condition, and retwist.

Shower Detangling

* Saturate your hair with water in the shower and divide it into two sections.
* Cleanse your hair with shampoo, one side at a time.
* Apply slippery conditioner to both sides in a smooshing motion.
* Pass head back under the shower stream for a moment for even distribution and added slip.
* Clip the hair up and out of the way while you complete showering.
* Take down the right side and detangle it (from the ends to the roots) under the water stream with your fingers or a shower comb or with a special detangling comb such as the Ouidad Double Detangler. Follow up

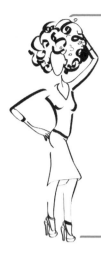

with the left side. If the conditioner is washed away
and tangles are left, add more conditioner and repeat.
The power of the water stream and the slip of the
conditioner should make detangling a breeze!

Damp Detangling

* Spritz dry hair with water and apply a conditioner or
  moisturizing butter to soften and add slip.
* Separate the hair into four to eight sections for easier
  handling.
* Choose a section and detangle gently with your
  fingers, moving from the ends to the roots, removing
  the knots and tangles.

    Optional: Comb through with a wide tooth comb or a
    paddle brush.
* Twist the section and move on to the next.
* Once you are in the shower, you can (1) shampoo and
  condition your hair in the twisted sections; (2) take

down all of the twists, being careful not to retangle your hair while washing and conditioning; or (3) take down one section at a time, shampoo, condition, and retwist.

Try each detangling method discussed here (modified to your needs and schedule) and see which works best. How will you know which one is for you? Trust me, it'll be obvious—excessive amounts of hair in the comb and hair blocking the shower drain are both red flags. You won't know what works until you experiment a bit. Try routines for a month, assess, and proceed from there.

LET'S GET PHYSICAL

When we're happy with our hair, our attention naturally drifts to other areas of our body that we could improve upon and some of us head to the gym. But exercise is not only great for your long-term health, it's also great for your hair health. Regular exercise is essential for healthy hair. It increases the oxygen in the blood circulating through your body, which provides an extra boost of oxygen to your hair's follicles and helps to accelerate its growth. A cardio workout stimulates circulation to your scalp, which promotes healthy hair growth as well. Exercising at least three times a week will make your hair healthy and shiny. Remember, your hair reflects the health of your body. Exercise and fuel it well, and your hair will grow, shine, and prosper.

How to Exercise and Maintain Gorgeous Hair

By Shelli Gillis

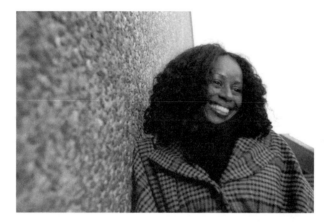

The primary deciding factor in my journey to natural was related to my exercise regimen. I was wearing my relaxed hair curly, because it was far easier to maintain than straight hair with a six-day-a-week workout schedule. Although natural hair may be easier to maintain than straight hair when one exercises regularly, it comes with its own unique set of challenges. However, there are some styles that can withstand sweaty routines more easily than others. There are also ways to be cute during your workout and to preserve your do postroutine.

STYLES

Protective styles, such as cornrows, flat twists, braids, two-strand twists, and mini-twists, are great for working out. They contain the hair to reduce frizzing, allow the scalp to breathe, and provide easy access for postworkout cleansing.

Buns are an elegant, quick, and versatile option that transitions seamlessly from the office to the gym. They can be sleek and professional but are also functional when you're working up a sweat, since they keep your hair off your perspiring neck and face. Think outside of the box when it comes to styling your hair. You can wear one bun or four. You can wear them braided, twisted, high, low, or to the side. There are so many styles from which to choose.

With the right preparation (see the next section), loose styles, such as braid-outs, twist-and-curls, and wash-and-gos, can also survive an intense workout and keep you looking cute at the same time.

PREWORKOUT PREP

When wearing braids or twists that hang on your neck and/or in your face, put them in a bun or a high ponytail. If your twists or braids are too short to fit into a scrunchie or form into a bun or a ponytail, simply secure them back and up, toward your crown, with bobby pins.

If loose styles are your preference, try piling the hair in a high, loose pineapple using a satin or silk scrunchie. [See Nikki's Perfect Pineapple instructions on page 117.] Or put your hair into two to six large braids or twists and secure them into buns or ponytails.

With any of these options, tie a satin or silk scarf around your hairline and wear a cotton bandana or a sweatband over it. The bandana or sweatband will absorb the sweat, and the silk/satin scarf will keep the hair smooth, as well as protect it from the moisture-robbing cotton of the bandana or sweatband.

If the scarf/bandana combo is not to your liking, you can try athletic headbands such as Dri Sweat Edge Women's Headband or Dri Sweat Active Wear Protector Cap, both by the Wave Enforcer.

POSTWORKOUT ROUTINE

Once you finish working out, remove the bandana or sweatband, but leave the satin or silk scarf on until your hair dries completely. This step is very important as it will reduce the possibility of excessive frizz.

Those without scalp concerns may be able to wash once a week or even less frequently. If you wear a wash-and-go and/or have scalp problems, you may need to shampoo with a sulfate-free shampoo or co-wash a few times a week. Try swabbing your scalp with an astringent like witch hazel or vinegar to remove sweat, dirt, and product buildup between wash sessions if you frequently experience an itchy, flaky scalp.

Nothing beats feeling healthy from head to toe!

Shelli Gillis has been wearing her hair in its natural state since 2000, when an overzealous stylist decided to put relaxer on more than her new growth. She big chopped well before she had ever heard of the term and she's been wearing her hair curly ever since. She started *Hairscapades,* her blog, at the encouragement of friends because she loves reading, writing, and talking about natural and curly hair.

exercise is good for your body and your mind!

Research shows that exercise is literally the best medicine for depression. It tops talk therapy and prescription meds by far. Unfortunately, it's often the last thing my clients want to do. They feel emotionally and physically drained and can barely drag themselves out of bed. But once they get up and moving, the motivation kicks in, as do the endorphins. Exercise is also great for preventing a relapse, so clients in recovery find it beneficial to keep exercising regularly. The psychological and physical benefits of exercise can also help reduce anxiety and improve mood. Whenever I'm stressed or feeling tired or sluggish for no reason, a brisk walk always helps.

It's also good for gaining confidence. Meeting exercise goals or challenges, even small ones, can boost your self-esteem. Getting in shape can also make you feel better about your appearance, which in turn helps with overall mood. So get your butt on a treadmill!

NIKKI RECOMMENDS HENNA

Nikki says: I began my henna journey in October 2007. I hennaed two to three times a week for the first month. After I read that henna has a cumulative effect (the more you do it, the more apparent the results), I went full steam ahead with it. I saw the color and shine after about two treatments, but the loosening, defrizzing, and even richer shine developed over several weeks. From November 2007 to January 2008, I hennaed once a week, or once every other week, and since then, I've been hennaing once a month. It can get to be a bit expensive, depending on the frequency of application, but it is so worth it!

My hair is shinier, *stronger,* and silkier. Henna has drastically decreased my breakage and splitting, reduced shrinkage, and has improved the overall look and health of my hair.

Picking the Perfect Henna

You can either buy henna from a reputable source online or at your local Indian grocer. Nikki uses and recommends several body art quality brands from Mehandi.com. If you go to an Indian grocer, buy body art quality henna only—none of that "blonde henna" or "black henna." Henna comes in one color: *red.* Make sure that the henna you buy looks fresh. It should be green, like spinach—but not a nuclear green because then it could have added dyes to make it *appear* fresh. It should smell earthy and not contain excessive grit, sticks, or sand. Henna should be a smooth, consistent powder that's easy to whip up, apply, and rinse out. A high quality, thoroughly sifted henna will rinse cleanly rather quickly. If you're still scratching leaves and twigs from your scalp days later, you need to switch brands. Nikki likes henna that leaves her gray hairs a dark copper after the first treatment. The second and third treatments will turn the copper color auburn.

Nikki's Henna Routine

Time needed: 12 hours
What you'll need:
    Newspaper
    150–200 grams body art quality Jamila Henna
        (www.mehandi.com)

1½–2 cups cooled green tea (brew 4 bags in filtered
  water)
A plastic tub with a lid (any old plastic container will do)
Conditioner
Honey
Plastic gloves
Plastic caps
Old satin scarf
Cotton balls
Moisturizing deep conditioner treatment

STEP 1 If you're a newbie at this and don't want what
will look like poop stains everywhere, lay down some
newspaper where you'll be working.

STEP 2 Mix your henna and green tea in the plastic tub
and put the lid on. Jamila Henna releases as you are
mixing it. But if you're using another type, you might
need to let it sit for anywhere from 20 minutes to 20
hours. Check the instructions.

STEP 3 Condition and detangle your hair, ideally in the
shower.

STEP 4 Once you get out of the shower, take the lid off
the henna mix and add about 3 tablespoons of honey to
make the mixture smoother and to aid in the rinsing
process.

STEP 5 With gloved hands, apply the pudding-like
mixture to small sections of your wet (but not dripping)
hair and put on a plastic cap. The henna will need to
be left on for 12 hours or so, so it's best to apply it on
a weekend night (around seven p.m.). To sleep in the

henna, don two plastic caps and a satin scarf that you won't mind getting dirty. If you start to leak, create a cotton ball barrier between the elastic of the cap and your skin.

STEP 6 When morning comes, you will most likely be excited to rinse the henna out of your hair and reveal your lovely tresses underneath. Fill the tub halfway with lukewarm water, get on your knees and dunk your head in. Splash around to loosen the hair up a bit, then position your head under the faucet and let the pressured water get most of the henna out.

STEP 7 Drain the tub, then promptly get back in the shower and turn on the shower head. While the water from the shower stream is cleaning out the tub, load your hair up with a ton of slippery conditioner, to soften it a bit. Then begin rinsing, and rinsing, and rinsing some more (upward of four times).

STEP 8 Apply a deep conditioner, add heat, and leave on for about an hour (see our deep conditioning treatment in chapter 2) before rinsing.

STEP 9 Now that your hair is looking glorious and supershiny, you're ready for a fetching hairstyle. I get the best, most-defined, and longest-lasting twist-outs after a henna treatment. I also get fuller-looking buns and protective styles.

Needless to say, after a henna weekend, everything on your body will be squeaky-clean! It's the perfect way to rejuvenate both your skin and hair.

Abbreviated Henna Treatment

Don't have time to spend 12 hours on your hair? Try this abbreviated version of the Nikki's henna treatment on dry hair.

Time needed: 6 hours
What you'll need:
- 2 cups water
- 1 tablespoon orange juice or apple cider vinegar or 2 bags green or chamomile tea
- Plastic or glass container
- 200 grams body art quality Jamila Henna (www.mehandi.com)
- Honey
- Wide tooth comb
- Plastic gloves
- Plastic caps
- Cotton balls
- Silk scarf
- Hooded hair dryer or micro heat cap
- Instant conditioner
- Moisturizing deep conditioner treatment

STEP 1 Whip up and apply the treatment (1 hour):
- * Bring the water to nearly boiling and remove from the heat.
- * Add the acid—either the orange juice or apple cider vinegar—to the water or, my personal favorite, add the tea bags to the water to brew.
- * In the plastic or glass container, mix the slightly acidic water or tea with the henna.

* Mix in 1 tablespoon (or more) of honey. The end result should look like thick mashed potatoes. It's okay if it's slightly runny, as it will make for an easier application. Cover the container and take it where you will apply the henna (most likely the bathroom).
* Gently detangle your dry hair with your fingers (you can follow up with the wide tooth comb if you like).
* Twist detangled sections (aim for eight to twelve twists).
* Put on a pair of plastic gloves, then clip all of the twists out of the way, except for the one you want to work with. (I always start in the back and work toward the front.)
* Take down the twist, and then apply the henna in a smooshing motion. Layer it on thick, like cake batter. Do not attempt to comb the henna through your hair.
* Repeat with the other twists.
* Gather up your hair and don a plastic cap, placing stretched-out cotton balls around the outer edge for comfort and to prevent the henna from dripping. Finally, throw on a pretty silk scarf so you don't scare your roommate or significant other.

STEP 2 Apply a heat source and allow your hair to marinate (4 hours or more):

* Sit under a hooded dryer or put on your micro heat cap on and off in 20-minute intervals for the next 4 hours.

The curl-loosening effect, caused by the weight of henna buildup, is most often experienced by naturals who have S-shaped waves, not coils. If you'd like to prevent this effect, add 2 tablespoons amla powder to your henna mix. This will help you retain your curl, but it will also push the henna's reddish color to more of a brown. Another option? Only henna your *roots* regularly, limiting full-head treatments to once every few months.

As with most hair treatments, henna may or may not be for you. Just because a product is "natural" doesn't mean it's all good. Try *patch testing*—hennaing a small patch at the back of your head—to ensure that you're not allergic and that you're comfortable with the color and texture of your hennaed hair. If you decide to start a henna regimen, do your research and listen to your hair every step of the way!

- or -

* You can go to sleep and allow your body heat to warm things up for 8 to 10 hours.

STEP 3 Rinse and apply a deep conditioner (1 hour or more):

* Run water in your tub, kneel over the tub, and dunk your head. Gently massage your hair and work the henna loose. Allow the water stream from the tub faucet to run through your hair, rinsing it clean. Apply a slippery conditioner and put your head back under the water stream. Repeat until your hair is henna-free.

* Pat your hair dry, section it, and apply a

moisturizing deep conditioning treatment.

* Don a clean plastic cap and apply a heat source
  for 15 to 30 minutes.
* Finally, jump in the shower, rinse your hair
  thoroughly, and style as usual.

Remember, four hours is the minimum amount of time that henna must be left on for you to reap its color and strengthening benefits. In fact, some argue that any longer than four hours is useless because you've already saturated your hair at that point. In an ideal world, if you plan to do a quick treatment, you would allow the henna mix to sit and release for a few hours prior to application. But if you're a busy mom flying by the seat of your pants like Nikki, just getting the opportunity to apply henna to your hair is better than nothing. And the heat will help it penetrate better.

Pros of the Abbreviated Henna Treatment vs. Nikki's Henna Routine

* Nearly the same results as the full treatment with
  much less time involved.
* Fewer (if any) drips, since you're applying the henna
  to dry hair.

Cons of the Abbreviated Henna Treatment vs. Nikki's Henna Routine

* Harder to rinse out the henna mixture (it's not as
  melted and pliable as it would be after sitting on your
  head for ten or more hours).

* Intense (applying and rinsing, deep treating, and styling all in one day!).

There's much debate as to whether henna dye uptake is more effective on dry as opposed to wet hair. Our feeling is that the results will be the same either way. Obviously, if your hair is difficult to detangle when it's dry, or is full of gel or has lots of buildup, hop in the shower and proceed with the wet application process. Remember, do what works for you.

Nikki's Henna Gloss Recipe

A henna gloss is used when you want subtle color change along with deep conditioning. It's easier to apply because of the wonderful slip provided by the conditioner. Since it's part conditioner and part henna, it's not a full-strength treatment. It's more like a deep conditioning treatment with some of the benefits of henna. You get much more moisture during the process, and it doesn't leave your hair as dry upon rinsing as a full henna treatment might do. This abbreviated henna treatment will leave your hair smooth and moisturized, not dry.

Be advised that this milder henna treatment will give you very little color change. You'll also miss out on the conditioning effects of a full-strength henna treatment. But this is a great option for two types of folks.

THOSE WHO WANT TO SEE WHAT THE HYPE IS ABOUT WITHOUT MAKING THE COLOR COMMITMENT. Henna is strong so be sure to do a strand test first. Mix 1 to 2 tablespoons henna directly into your conditioner (not allowing for dye release) and leave it in your hair for 20 to 30 minutes only. Be forewarned: the henna may still leave behind a red tint.

FAITHFUL HENNAERS WHO WANT TO EXPERIENCE SOFT, SMOOTH HAIR UPON RINSING. It's truly amazing! You'll hopefully be left with a similar dye release, color uptake, strengthening, and smoothing. After a henna gloss your hair is soft and smooth immediately upon rinsing, even before the deep conditioning step. A henna gloss essentially combines the henna and deep conditioning steps.

What you'll need:
- 1½ cups water
- 1 tablespoon orange juice or apple cider vinegar or 2 bags green or chamomile tea
- Plastic or glass container
- At least 100 grams body art quality Jamila Henna (www.mehandi.com)
- Light, protein-free conditioner (we suggest GVP Conditioning Balm, which is the generic version of Matrix Biolage Conditioning Balm, available at Sally Beauty; see the appendix for more ideas)
- Plastic cap
- Cotton balls or tissue
- Scarf
- Moisturizing deep conditioner treatment (or honey and unsweetened yogurt)

STEP 1 Mix the henna as you would for a regular, full-strength treatment. Nikki adds 100 grams Jamila Henna to 1½ cups warm green tea. (She never measures. She just gets it to the consistency of cake batter.)

STEP 2 Mix in 1 cup of the conditioner.

STEP 3 Apply the henna-conditioner mixture to your dry or damp and detangled hair in sections. Then don a plastic cap and insert cotton balls or rolled-up tissues near your ears to catch drips. Put a scarf on top.

STEP 4 Leave in the henna mixture for the desired amount of time. Remember, the shorter the time (15 to 30 minutes), the less dye uptake, which means less red but also less conditioning. If you leave it in overnight, you'll get the full benefits of henna with the added bonus of a moisturizing deep conditioning treatment.

STEP 5 Dunk your head under the tub faucet to wash away most of the henna mixture. Hop in the shower and rinse away the rest using a slippery conditioner. (Note that the henna mixture will rinse very easily, so you can probably skip washing your hair under the faucet.)

STEP 6 Do a deep conditioning treatment, using honey and yogurt, if desired. (Some women use yogurt in place of conditioner.)

STEP 7 Rinse and style your hair as usual.

REMEMBER . . .

* You can modify this recipe and leave the henna-conditioner mixture in for less time if you want only a subtle color change. If you want the full benefits of

color and henna's conditioning powers, leave it in for at least 4 hours or overnight.

* Use a conditioner free of protein and preferably free of silicones.
* If you're trying this mixture, use the least amount of tea possible. Use too much and you'll have an annoying, runny mess.

Using Henna to Cover Gray Hair

Nikki suggests a henna with a high dye content such as Jamila, which may be purchased at Mehandi.com, for coloring your gray roots. Jamila Henna has a very high dye content (3.4 percent lawsone) and yields a deep auburn color over time. Remember that multiple applications will be necessary for your gray hair to darken to the color you want. But over time, your gray hair will become a rich auburn color (gorgeous!), and the rest of your hair will be fuller, shinier, and healthier looking. Your hair will be a rich, shiny black color indoors (with a few red highlights) and glow auburn in the sun.

When new gray hairs come in or your roots show, simply apply an overnight treatment, and after a couple of days, your gray hair will oxidize to a nice bronzy red. After another treatment, the roots will be the same color as your auburn length.

For those trying to cover their gray hair, the keys to success will be:

1. Four-hour (or longer) treatments.
2. Multiple applications (for darker results).
3. Cleansing prior to application. If you have a lot of

gray hair, this step is crucial. It will remove buildup and sebum (a fatty skin secretion) so that the dye can make the best contact with your roots.

Also, be sure to condition a lot afterward to keep your hair moisturized, elastic, and supple.

What Henna *Won't Do*

* Henna won't lighten your hair.
* If your hair is black, henna won't provide a full-on color change. It sounds weird, but the color of your hennaed hair will change depending on the setting. It's sort of like a rinse, a transparent coppery rinse. Imagine drawing with an orange crayon on black construction paper. Under most indoor lighting, the paper still looks black (albeit shinier), but if held under the light a certain way, you'll catch a glimpse of orange. Outdoors in sunlight Nikki's hair glows auburn, so much so that her sister and husband call her "redhead," but indoors it's a rich black. There are some instances (back lighting, etc.) where you can really see the red indoors, but she has never been able to catch the color on camera.
* If your hair is lighter (e.g., sandy brown), the red will be very evident. Your hair may appear auburn in most lighting conditions.
* Henna won't stop damaged hair from breaking or splitting. It will not mend split ends—nothing will. Henna will, however, fortify your strands, reduce breakage, and prevent the damage that causes split

ends in the first place. It mimics a protein treatment, which is why you must use a moisturizing conditioner immediately following a henna application to keep your hair soft and pliable.

CUTTING YOUR OWN HAIR

In order for your natural hair to truly thrive, you must be vigilant about keeping it free of split ends. Split ends not only look bad but can also hinder your hair growth by catching on adjacent (and usually healthy or split-free) hairs and causing tangles and matting that can lead to more splits and breakage during the detangling process.

You can tell if an end is damaged because it looks jagged (instead of tapered) or looks torn, has a white dot (which means it broke off at that point, most likely from heat damage), or is split in two or, worse, three hairs. Examine your ends in good lighting. Also, if detangling has become more difficult than usual as of late, you could probably use a trim.

But there's no need to hit the salon every time you spot a split end. "Dusting" your hair every two months is a great way to keep your ends neat and free of split ends.

STEP 1 Twist your hair. It's best to opt for eight to ten twists, as it's easier to keep your hair even if you cut it in larger sections.

STEP 2 Survey the end of each twist. Snip off the last ⅛ to ¼ inch. Trim depending on the state of your ends and how long it's been since the last trim.

dusting \dəst-tin\

[noun]

A micro-trimming technique that is performed on twisted hair.

STEP 3 Moisturize and oil each twist as you go. Seal the ends with a water-based conditioner or moisturizer (one that's not too thick), such as one by Elucence (www .elucence.com) or Star Lacio Lacio High Shine Leave-in Conditioner, and seal the twist with an oil mix (castor oil plus jojoba oil if you're feeling organic or a silicone serum if you're feeling randy).

In between dusting sessions, consider conducting "search and destroy" missions to keep your ends sharp. Just grab a curl while sitting in front of the TV, standing in front of the bathroom mirror, or even while on the Internet and inspect it for split ends. If you find any, you can snip them on the spot.

But if you're too busy or your hair is too short to do these checks, schedule it on your calendar for every two months and dust accordingly. Remember, an ounce of prevention . . .

FABULOUS SECOND-DAY HAIR

Curlfriends are always in search of that elusive "second-day hair"—a style that lasts forty-eight hours and still looks fab! Here's the thing: achieving dependable second-, third-, or fourth-day hair takes preparation, starting with a solid, moisture-based regimen on wash day, followed by protective measures at night, and, if necessary, some refreshing the morning after. Here's how.

MOISTURIZE. Properly moisturized curls retain their definition and ward off frizz. On wash day, use a gentle, nonstripping shampoo, deep condition with heat, use a leave-in conditioner, and follow up with an oil to seal in all that moisture.

Tip: Apply your leave-in and oil in a downward motion to smooth the cuticle, and in small sections, to ensure it's evenly and thoroughly distributed.

SET. Many curlfriends find that their curls last longer if they have the "crunch factor" from a styling gel or cream on day one. A firm-hold product locks in the curls, resulting in a "perfect" and less voluminous look, which will slowly loosen and fluff up over time. If you choose this route, apply the styler after your leave-in and oil. When buying your styler, look for aloe vera gel in the ingredients list as it encourages definition and provides moisture.

Tip: Once your hair is styled, don't touch it or you'll risk major frizz! You have to allow your style and curls to properly set.

PROTECT. "Pineappling" (see page 118), or gathering your curls in a high, loose ponytail, will keep your curls from shrinking, flattening, and frizzing. If your hair is

NIKKI'S PERFECT PINEAPPLE

Nikki says: This is my nighttime "pineapple" routine for whenever I need to get second- or third-day hair. You can pineapple whenever you want to try to preserve your curls for the next day, so they don't get smooshed and frizzy while you sleep. And since you're only loosely gathering your hair, it's not damaging. Top off the pineapple with a bonnet (extra protection!) and you're good to go.

What you'll need:
A satin scrunchie (I like scrunchies because they don't leave indentations in your hair.)

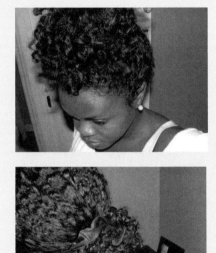

STEP 1   Bend over at the waist and loosely gather your hair at the crown of your head. Pull your hair through the scrunchie twice to make it secure but not tight.

STEP 2   Then it's off to bed.

STEP 3 The next morning, take down your hair and shake it vigorously. If your hair's temperament is similar to mine, it would be perfectly happy standing up in a Don King–esque style and may need to be coaxed back down. Use the same scrunchie to gather your hair at the nape of your neck while you eat breakfast, shower, and dress for the day. Before you head out the door, remove the scrunchie and shake your hair out. This last step helps for when you've slept with your hair out, too.

The key to a good pineapple is to keep the scrunchie loose. A too-tight scrunchie could lead to flat, stretched-out, sad-looking curls. Trust us!

short, you can try a low, loose ponytail or multiple loose ponytails. Other naturals find retwisting, rebraiding, or doing a bun to be a better method of curl preservation.

Tip: No matter how you style your hair at bedtime, everyone should cover her hair with a satin or silk bonnet and sleep on a satin-covered pillow.

REVIVE. Even with preparation, our curls can be a bit unpredictable. Salvage your style by coating the frizzy pieces with a leave-in conditioner-water mix, finger curling and twisting the flattened pieces, or spritzing your hair with a mix of water, aloe vera gel, and oil.

Tip: If all else fails, you can always rock a fierce updo (more on updos later in the chapter).

TRAVELING WHILE CURLY

One of the most-talked-about benefits of going natural is the ability to truly enjoy your vacations. No more roasting away on the beach because you're afraid of what the ocean will do to your hair, and when you get hit with a tropical shower, you

Your Best Curlfriend Says . . .

Don't want a standard black satin pillowcase? Try JCPenney or Amazon.com for nonstandard sizes and a bigger color selection.

can feel free to frolic in the rain as opposed to high-tailing it to the nearest covered shelter. Many of our curlfriends report that they decided to big chop before a vacation so that they could actually enjoy their fun in the sun without any hair anxiety. Here are a few of our favorite dos and don'ts for traveling while curly.

DO wear a protective style on the plane. Everyone knows that airplane cabins are super-dehydrating. Do your hair a favor by deep conditioning, moisturizing, and putting it in a protective style before you head out. Drink lots of water on the plane and take down your hair when you get to your destination. Or even better, if you really want a no-fuss vacation, put your hair in a protective style like braids or twists and don't mess with it, except to spritz as needed with a diluted leave-in conditioner-water mix, for the rest of the vacation.

DON'T fight nature. Don't waste your valuable vacation time prepping for a style that may or may not work in heavy humidity. Instead, opt for wash-and-gos, buns, braids, and twists. Also, keep one of those superchic, oversized sun hats for days when you don't want to be bothered dealing with your hair.

DO pack on the protein. Nicole Harmon, the wise cosmetic chemist from the *Hair Liberty* blog, once told us, "Products that contain hydrolyzed protein temporarily patch up some of the cuticle holes in porous hair. If African American hair doesn't get additional protein regularly, it will frizz out very quickly no matter what you do." If you're traveling to or live in a humid climate, regularly use products that contain hydrolyzed proteins. Also, look for products that contain silicones (amodimethicone) and polymers (PVP/VA copolymer) in the first five ingredients. These ingredients help to create a barrier on your strands, locking in moisture from your conditioner and locking out moisture from the atmosphere.

DON'T try out new styles—especially if you're traveling for business. Save yourself the anxiety of a disastrous hairstyle gone wrong by sticking to the styles you know when you travel. Also, pack plenty of extra decorative or simple side combs, headbands, and hair accessories, just in case even your go-to style lets you down.

DO protect your hair before swimming. Harmon recommends that you rinse your hair with tap water prior to entering the pool. If your hair is "filled up" with tap water, it will absorb less of the chlorinated water (a wet sponge has a difficult time soaking up more water). Next, apply a coating of conditioner or a silicone serum to further hinder the chlorinated water's ability to seep into your strands. Then, don a sexy swim cap (just be careful that it doesn't pull at your hairline). Once your pool fun is done, shampoo with a cleanser designed to rid your strands of chlorine (pick up a shampoo designed to do this at your local beauty-supply store). Then deep condition and style as usual.

DON'T leave behind your staple products just because they don't come in travel sizes. Decide what cleanser, detangling conditioner, moisturizer, sealant, and styler you would want with you on a desert island, and if they don't come in travel size, get the appropriate containers for them at your nearest drugstore. It helps if your favorite conditioner can work double duty—as a detangler in the shower and a leave-in for moisturizing.

JAZZING UP YOUR LOOK WHEN THE GOLDEN RAINBOW ISN'T ENOUGH

When we first begin our natural hair journey, many of us are obsessed with length—especially if our journey begins with a big chop. We can't wait to look like the women in our next chapter, the ones with long, natural hair, the ones who never have to fret that their hair is too short to do that amazing updo we just saw on YouTube.

However, once you've achieved good to dramatic lengths, you might find yourself growing bored with the whole endeavor if you don't find ways to keep yourself occupied on your multiyear journey. That's where a different style might come in handy. Here are a few ways to perk up your golden look.

Simple Changes

If you're a wash-and-go girl, try a twist-out. If you're a twist-out girl, try a roller set for loose curls or Curlformers for a press and curl look.

How to Get a Delicious Afro Without Heat

By TiaShauntee

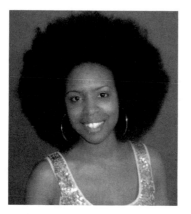

Before doing any type of blow out/ afro hairstyle, make sure to pamper you hair. Pre-poo, shampoo, deep condition, and detangle *well*. Start with stretched hair (hair you've either braided or twisted the night before) so that you'll get the biggest afro possible. If you start on hair that isn't stretched, your afro will appear smaller and more compact.

STEP 1 Pick out your hair into the shape that you want your afro.

STEP 2 Once your hair is picked out, mist it lightly with water and let shrinkage do its thing. It's key that you refrain from touching your hair as much as possible during this step because your hair will lose the shape you've picked out. Only touch your hair in order to maintain and shape your afro. And voilà, you have a delicious afro without using heat.

If the luster has fallen off the natural hair movement for you, why not blow out your hair and try some vintage styles from the sixties and seventies. You can find some really clever ones at *Ebony* magazine Tumblr, Pinterest, and specialty sites such as Vintage Black Glamour. But before you attempt any of them, make sure to read the following section where we tell you how to make an afro without exposing your hair to heat damage. No one wants to end up looking like Mufasa.

You can also flat-iron your hair and try out some of the funkier styles you've seen featured in the latest *Essence* issue. One of the best things about having natural hair is its versatility. You can wear your hair straight for a wedding one day and go back to kinky curls the next, so do take advantage of your hair's malleability.

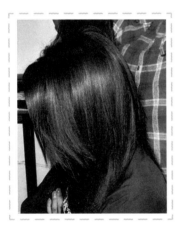

How to Safely Flat-Iron Your Hair

* Cleanse *thoroughly* (for straightening, use shampoo, not a cleansing conditioner), condition, and deep condition for 30 minutes with a gentle heat source.
* Apply a light coating of leave-in conditioner and/or oil (to lock in the moisture). We recommend these leave-in conditioners for straightening: Salerm 21, Star Lacio Lacio High Shine Leave-in Conditioner, and Redken Extreme Anti Snap. Make sure that whatever leave-in you choose contains protein. Although nothing can prevent all damage if you habitually straighten your hair, a good leave-in will fortify your strands, minimizing breakage.
* Apply a heat protectant such as Sabino Lok & Blok,

Redken Smooth Down Heat Glide Protective Smoother, or Fantasia IC Polisher Heat Protector Straightening Serum.

* Skip the blow-dryer. Instead, do chunky braids or roller set your hair to stretch it. Then air-dry overnight or sit under a bonnet dryer.

* If you must blow-dry, blot excess moisture and allow your hair to air-dry for 15 minutes prior to starting. Blow-drying wet hair can lead to a loss of elasticity and, in the long run, breakage. Keep the heat setting as low as possible and hold the nozzle a few inches away from your hair.

* Flat-iron your hair in *very* small sections with a ceramic-plated iron using the chase method: Detangle each section thoroughly with a wide tooth comb, then grab a comb with closer teeth and comb your hair from the roots down, just enough for the flat iron to fit between your roots and the comb, and "chase" the comb with the flat iron on the way down to your ends. The comb should always be above the iron. The tension provided by the comb should only make one pass necessary to get your hair its straightest.

* Keep the temperature of the flat iron as low as possible. Start on a cool setting and go up incrementally (by five degrees, if possible) until you reach an effective temperature. The straighter you get your hair in the stretching process, the less heat you'll need while flat-ironing. We recommend 300 to 350 degrees Fahrenheit, but nothing over 400.

* Finally, no touch-ups! When your hair is beginning to revert, bantu knot or twist it to achieve a wave pattern. Never flat-iron dirty hair. And sleep in a satin cap at night.

You might also want to try a funky braided style or a twisted updo. Although if you're like most of us, you'll have to get professional help to achieve the more complicated styles featured in magazines and online. Most truly funky styles are best handled by a professional, unless you want to put in hours learning how to braid, cut, and apply color to your own hair. Here are some of our favorite looks to try with a hairstylist.

Coloring

In general, we advise against coloring your hair with anything stronger than henna because permanent and temporary dyes make your hair prone to breakage, splitting, and chronic dryness. But if a lighter color or highlights are just *calling* to you, make sure to get the coloring done by a professional. Don't use one of those at-home kits or you might end up with more hair

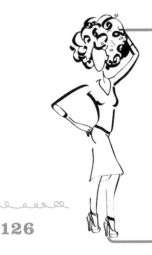

Your Best Curlfriend Says . . .

After you color, consider ditching the shampoo and switching to a co-washing regimen. Also, commit to deep conditioning weekly and using a daily leave-in. Your hair will need all the moisture it can get.

damage than the color is worth. Visit the CurlyNikki forums and ask around about stylists in your area who are good with both styling *and* coloring natural hair. Not every stylist can do both well.

Colored Extensions

While we don't highly recommend coloring your hair, we're crazy about colored extensions. If done well, they can make even the most rudimentary twist-out go from boring to popping. Just make sure you don't keep them in for more than six weeks or they might end up popping *and* locking, forcing you to cut them out. Also, ask your hairstylist to braid in your natural extensions as opposed to using glue, which can damage the hair shaft, irritate the scalp, and rip out your natural hair when removed. Braiding is much less harmful to your hair and scalp, not to mention much easier to take out yourself.

A Bold Cut

If you're not attached to length, then you might be the perfect candidate for a creative cut. Instead of a fauxhawk, you can try a real frohawk with your hair shaven at the sides. Or you can try something similar to what our very cool curlfriend Chime Edwards (aka HairCrush) did. She shaved one side of her head but still has the ability to flip her hair over to hide it if she wishes. Talk to your stylist about asymmetrical cuts, and always keep in mind your hair's awesome versatility. If you see it, you can probably achieve it with the help of a hairstylist.

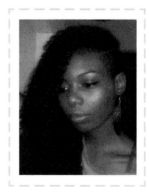

Step Up Your Protective Style!

By Charnika "CharyJay" Jett

At month nine in my transitioning journey, and after constant manipulation of my hair, my ends were almost nonexistent. After hearing about how protective styles can help retain length and protect your hair against the elements, I thought that just maybe these kinds of styles could salvage the ends I had left.

I had absolutely no flat-twisting or braiding skills, so I decided to practice those styles, and after about two weeks of epic failed attempts, I had a semi-decent style that was good enough to see the light of day. To my surprise it got a lot of compliments, and while I don't count on others' comments to make myself feel good about my hair, it gave me the confidence to try more styles.

With each attempt, my flat-twisting improved and so did the health of my hair. No more crazy amounts of shedded hair on my clothes, hours dedicated to detangling sessions, or a requirement to do my hair two to three times a week. No ma'am, protective styling seemed to cure all of those problems, and it came with one added bonus: it helped me feed into my creative side as well.

I started to challenge myself to see what style I could come up with next. *How creative can you get today?* It was almost like a contest I had with my last style. *Which one would win?* It was a lot of fun then and it still is now.

Styling my hair means even more to me at this point because I can inspire others to step outside of their comfort zone and try something different with their hair. We can all get bored doing the same "old faithful style" every time wash day comes along, and

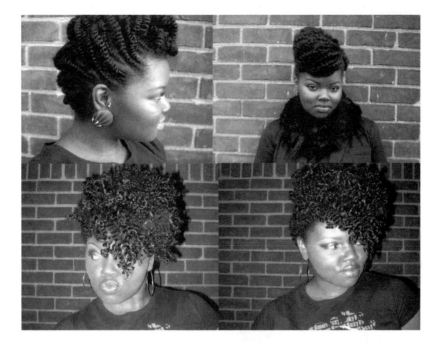

sometimes we just need something different to inspire us and take ourselves and our hair to the next level. So many women have seen a look I did and created something totally different and made it their own. That's what it's all about! Getting creative with your hair and making it work for you.

I started doing protective styles because my hair absolutely needed it. Now, my hair is as healthy as ever and I'm still doing them. Not because it's a necessity for the overall health of my hair, but for my love and passion for haute hairstyles that anyone can make work for themselves.

Charnika Jett is a journalist and videographer who resides in Detroit, Michigan. When she's not working, she loves to travel around the world to different natural hair meet-ups. There she shares her knowledge and offers support and encouragement to those women who are already natural or are thinking about going natural.

GOLDEN UPDOS FOR WORK, WEEKEND, AND GLAMOROUS EVENTS

Mane and Chic's Southern Tease Bun

STEP 1 Gather and smooth your dry, detangled hair at the nape of your neck.

STEP 2 Gently twist so that your hair ends form a tip.

STEP 3 Place the tip (ends of your hair) to the back of your head.

STEP 4 Now grab the hair on the right side and pull it to the middle to hide the tip.

STEP 5 Grab the hair on the left side and pull it to the middle to meet the hair from the right side.

STEP 6 Secure your hair with a large bobby pin.

This style is low manipulation and takes about 5 seconds to do. There are no elastics involved, which means even less stress on your curls. Nikki calls it her go-to Mom Bun. Adorn with a flower and/or leave some hair loose in the front to frame your face.

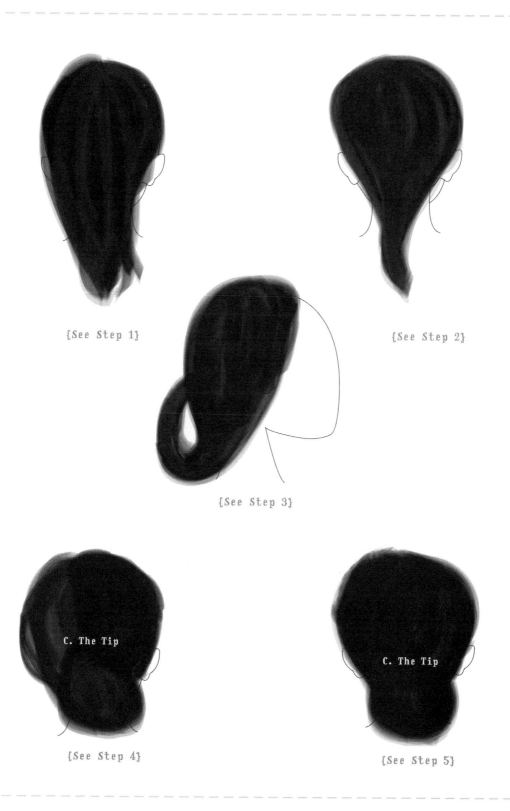

{See Step 1}

{See Step 2}

{See Step 3}

C. The Tip

{See Step 4}

C. The Tip

{See Step 5}

Bun and Pomp

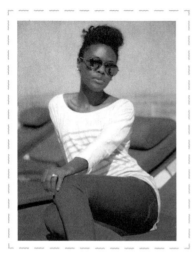

STEP 1 With dry hair, section off some bangs and pin it out of the way.

STEP 2 Gather the rest of your hair and create a bun— high, low, on the side, anywhere! You can use an elastic band (no metal on it) to secure your bun, pulling the hair through twice and only halfway through the third time.

-or-

You can free-form the bun using bobby pins, tucking and pinning your hair appropriately.

STEP 3 Fluff the bangs, lightly twist the end, and secure it with bobby pins so that it stands up. Use shea butter or a light gel to smooth your edges on the side for a sleeker look.

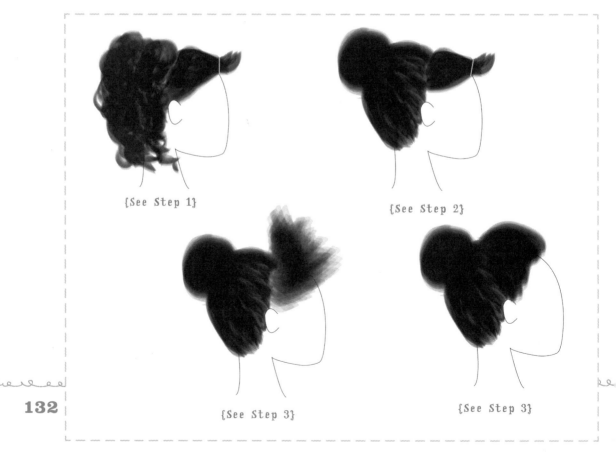

{See Step 1}

{See Step 2}

{See Step 3}

{See Step 3}

High Side Bun with Headband

To get this look, simply pull dry hair (preferably a fresh twist-out) up near the crown of your head but off center. Adorn with a cute headband. Instant glam and perfect for travel!

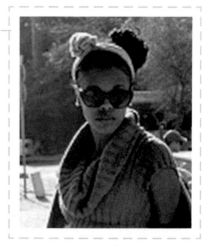

Supereasy and Elegant Twist-and-Curl Fauxhawk

Shelli Gillis of the blog *Hairscapades* uses a Goody banana clip to secure her fresh twist-and-curl into a cute fauxhawk. This style is perfect for work, fun, or a glamorous midweek event. Simply do a twist-and-curl on wash day and pull out the banana clip later in the week for instant glamour.

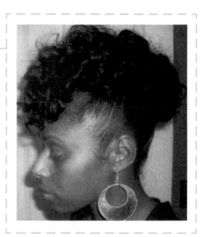

Figure 8 Bun and Pomp

Instructions provided by Danielle Faust from the blog OK, Dani.

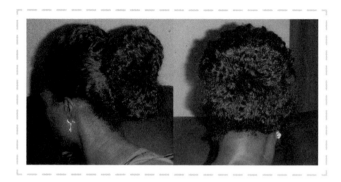

STEP 1 Start with a dry twist-out. Moisturize your hair with a lotion and an oil. Danielle used Silk Elements MegaSilk Leave-In Hair Moisturizing Creme and coconut oil to achieve this look.

STEP 2 Grab a small front section of hair and make and pin a pomp (see "Bun and Pomp" on page 132 for instructions).

STEP 3 Wrangle the rest of your hair into a ponytail, neither too low nor superhigh.

STEP 4 Split the ponytail into two pieces horizontally. (Meaning you have a top and a bottom section, not a left and a right section.)

STEP 5 Roll the top section of the split ponytail upward into a lump and secure with bobby pins.

STEP 6 Roll the bottom section of the split ponytail downward into a lump and secure with bobby pins.

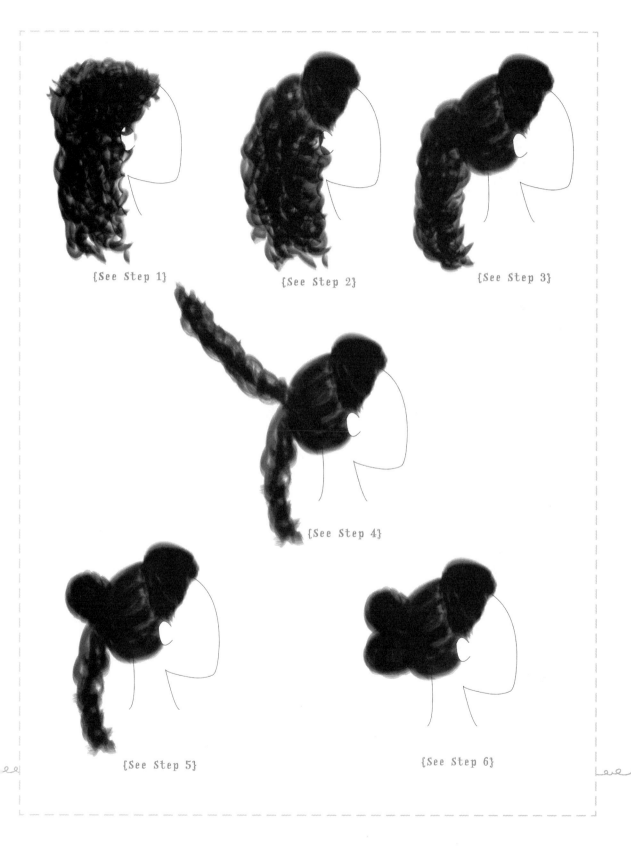

{See Step 1}

{See Step 2}

{See Step 3}

{See Step 4}

{See Step 5}

{See Step 6}

GOLDEN NATURALS SOUND OFF!

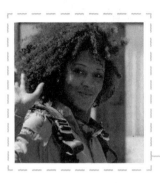

I love my natural hair because it is so versatile! I can wear it in two-strand twists, flat twist-outs, blow outs, and bantu knots. I have come to love my hair and accept it as part of my identity. The journey to this point has been tough, but I learned that if I am determined to do something, I will stick with it and succeed!

—Erica James

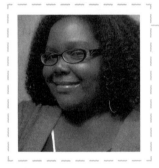

I work at a zoo, literally, and every day is an adventure. Having natural hair helps me not to be worried about whether it is going to rain when I am out with my animals, or if something gets into my hair. I can pull my hair in a bun and go about my day with little to no problems. I have curly girls who come up to me and say they love my hair and can't wait for their length to be the same as mine. I tell them I remember being in their shoes and to relax and enjoy the ride. My favorite day was when a little girl about eight years old came up to me while I was at work and said, "You have the same hair as mine! People make fun of my hair, but now I can say a zookeeper has the same hair as me!" Who doesn't love that?

—Desiree Brandon

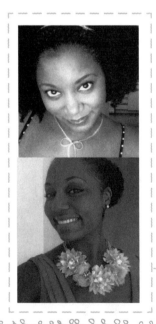

The process has been laborious at times, but I wouldn't change it for the world. I've been able to convince five friends to take the leap. It's important to me to spread the wealth of knowledge I've obtained regarding natural hair maintenance and growth. Black women can have beautiful tresses as long as we take care of what's been given to us.

—Brandi Preston

CHAPTER FIVE

Natural from the Start

Curly Kids

Just a few generations back, kinky hair was considered "unmanageable." Boys had their hair lopped off as soon as they were old enough to sit up by themselves in a barber chair, and girls with more than a few inches of hair quickly got introduced to a hot comb—much to the dismay of their poor burnt ears. In recent years, the age at which girls get their first perms has gotten younger and younger, and it's not uncommon these days to see even toddlers with relaxed hair. We're not going to get into

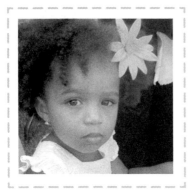

an argument about whether it's healthy to expose children to harsh chemicals at such a young age. That topic has been covered in other venues quite well, and we're not here to judge other mothers.

However, we do love that the natural hair movement has provided many mothers all over the world with a great alternative to relaxers and hot combs. And the even better news is that you don't have to be or become a braiding expert in order to keep your child's natural hair looking great. Today, there are lots of great options for taking care of your child's hair; so many, in fact, that you might be a little stymied figuring out which styling option is best for you. Here's our advice.

PROTECTIVE STYLING is the best option if you are busy or short on patience, or if you have a squirmy child. What's great about protective styles is that you only have to update them once or twice a week. "If I had it to do all over again today, I would just braid my girls' hair and call it a day," says fashion blogger Tenisha Mercer from *The Hairnista Chronicles*. "You know how day cares always tell you to dress your kids in 'play' clothes? Same thing with the hair. While I know intricate styles are beautiful, they may be a waste of time for younger girls. Braided hair is a good protective style that can withstand most of what your daughter or son is doing in day care and you won't have to manipulate it daily."

Braids and other protective styles are perfect for moms and children on the go. Some of our favorite protective styles include cornrows, box braids, two-strand twists, French rolls, buns, and the timeless classic two French braids.

MORNING STYLING is a great option if you have the time to spare or have a squirmy child. It seems counterintuitive to do daily styling on a child who won't sit still, but after the first few brutal weeks, you'll probably find that your child will respond to the consistency of the routine. She'll eventually stop fighting you, because it will become part of her morning. Morning styling is also great because it means that you can style your child's hair according to your energy level and any events coming up that day.

Morning styling is a fantastic option for mothers of children whose hair might not respond to protective styling. Ernessa has a biracial daughter whose hair just laughs at most protective styles. She's learned that it's easier to put her daughter's hair into a simple style in the morning before sending her off to preschool.

Your Mom Curlfriend Says . . .

Set aside a specific time every week to put your child's hair in a protective style.

you are not your child's hair

The state of your child's hair is not a visual representation of your mothering abilities. Kids will be kids, and if your daughter is anything like mine, her cute little braids are undone and turned into one massive, frizzy afro by day's end. I let her hair "do what it do," and I've caught flak from the old school women in my family. But I'm not going to stress myself over her hair. Kids are little sponges and are much more aware than we give them credit for. I never want Gia to think her hair stresses me out or that it's a source of frustration for me. Wouldn't it be a beautiful world if our daughters could be free of all the hang-ups we had with our hair growing up? Help them view their natural hair as beautiful and perfect just the way it grows. Teach them early that they already have better than good hair!

Some of our favorite cute-but-easy morning styles include double puffs with a straight or zigzag part, French braids, the single puff, and an afro with side combs. The last one is especially great if your child is in day care because it will stand up to hard play and nap time, and the end-of-the-day frizzy version of it still looks pretty good.

CUT IT ALL OFF if you're busy or have a squirmy child. We're including this option just to remind you that it is an option for girls as well as boys. Keeping your daughter's hair short before she's old enough to have her own hair preferences won't scar her for life.

And it's also the easiest option of those we've listed. If you're worried about her looking like a boy, use headbands and clothing to highlight her girliness.

TAKE YOUR CHILD TO A STYLIST if you're superbusy, you can afford it, and your child isn't squirmy. If your child can sit calmly for over an hour while someone does her or his hair, we're so jealous! Feel free to take advantage of this magical ability to sit still and outsource your hair duties to someone else. A professional braider can save you time by putting your daughter's or son's hair in a style that can last up to a month.

No matter what you decide to do with your child's hair, keep in mind that until she can start making a few hair decisions on her own, her hair duties are an extension of yours. If you don't have the energy to do your own hair every single morning, don't feel obligated to do more for your child than you would do for yourself. Experiment with different styles until you find a few go-to styles that work for both you and your child.

HAIR SQUIRM BUSTERS

Ask any mom. The number one enemy of a supercute style is your own squirmy child. Some children are perfect angels and will sit still on command for as long as it takes for you to do their hair. Congratulations, if that's your kid. For the

(Mostly) Drama-Free Hair Wash Days

By Nadine Afia

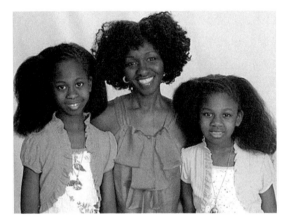

It was another standoff. I was chasing the younger of my two daughters around the sofa, determined to finish the postwash detangling session that she had abruptly abandoned in protest. It was a battle of wills, and one of us would eventually break.

Unfortunately, that "one of us" was usually me. There had to be a better way! It was frustrating moments like these that would bring back my own childhood hair memories.

When I was a child, the words "hair wash day" were guaranteed to strike the fear of God into me. I'm sure most children with parents of African descent can relate. At our house, hair wash day was executed like a military operation. Four girls meant four heads full of kinky, coily hair. This mission was not for the faint of heart. My mother was a warrior, and her weapons of choice were an industrial-size tub of Vaseline, a fresh bar of Lux bath soap (which could dry out an oil spill), an afro comb, and, for thorough detangling (shudders)—a rat tail comb. My sisters and I would stand at the bathroom door, eyes wide, as we watched the carnage. My mother was swift and focused. The wailing cries of her girls, with soap-stung eyes, did nothing to detract her from her mission. Her battle cry was "It hurts to be pretty!" I'll spare you the details of the rat tail comb detangling portion of this operation. But I assure you, "pretty" it was not.

Admittedly, once she had finished, our beautifully manicured tresses were a sight to behold: African-threaded styles, adorned with pretty barrettes and bows. Our afros and puffs would elicit oohs and aahs from passersby, and we would beam with pride.

Fast-forward to the present, and thankfully there are now so many helpful resources online, such as CurlyNikki and YouTube, where parents can learn, ask questions, and trade war stories. Whatever your child's hair type or texture, there's always someone with a tip or a trick that will help. Thanks to the Internet, and a little trial and error, I've discovered tear-free hair washing, detangling, and styling techniques. I also utilize the classic African-threading technique, used by my mother, to keep my daughters' hair stretched and tangle-free.

If my mother were here today, I know she'd be proud and amazed at how I've combined the traditional art of African threading with modern hair care techniques and hairstyles that result in (mostly) drama-free hair wash days.

- -

Nadine Afia, the mother of three, is a children's natural hair advocate whose informative and humorous YouTube channel, "GirlsLoveYourCurls," offers hair care and styling tips for kids. "GirlsLoveYourCurls" is a popular resource for parents who want their children to embrace their beautiful kinks and coils.

rest of us, here are some tips for dealing with a squirmy hair stylee.

CHOOSE THE RIGHT TIME. Protective styles can be done at any time of the day, so why attempt one when your child is wide awake with plenty of energy to battle your rat tail comb? Many of our curlfriends suggest putting in protective styles toward the end of the day, when your child is ~~too tired to fight you off~~ willing to veg out in front of the television while you go to work on that head. In fact . . .

BEDTIME MIGHT BE THE RIGHT TIME. A few of our curlfriends have reported pulling off a protective style while their children are sound asleep. If your child plays *and* sleeps hard, this might be the perfect time to put in those flat-strand twists!

BATH-TIME HAIR SALON. Get your two-strand twists on while your child relaxes in the bathtub with her rubber duckies.

TELEVISION IS YOUR COSTYLIST. Consider making television time hair time. Note your child's favorite video and only let her watch it during hair time. The television can also be used as a bribe. If your child doesn't sit still, then the television goes off. You'd be surprised how many children magically figure out how to stay in one place when doing so is connected to their favorite cartoon.

Your Mom Curlfriend Says . . .

If your child is tender-headed, make sure to hold the hair at the root while detangling or styling to reduce pulling. Detangling conditioners and/or oils will aid in the detangling process as well. Whether it's detangling or styling, have patience and only tackle small sections at a time. Finally, it's even more important to always opt for wide tooth, seamless combs with tender-headed children.

USE THE HIGH CHAIR. Who says high chairs are just for eating? Keep your child in the chair, and throw in a couple of afro puffs after breakfast while she's still strapped in.

TALKING WITH YOUR CHILDREN ABOUT RELAXERS

Nikki says: When I was a kid, relaxers weren't allowed in my home; it was very difficult at times—it didn't feel fair. I saw the girls with relaxed hair as having better styling options and straighter, thus prettier, hair. I would get very frustrated that the slightest bit of water would turn my press and curl into a puff ball.

I think learning styles that actually worked with my

texture as opposed to against it would have helped me tremendously back then. In my house, straight hair was seen as "appropriate" and thus my mom kept our hair pressed. Whenever it reverted, I felt ugly. I was never explicitly taught that my natural hair was ugly, I just learned from watching those close to me that straight hair was "professional," "neat," and "groomed." I think that if we'd explored other styles, such as twist-outs and braid-outs, afro puffs, and so on, it would've been easier to embrace my hair.

Here are some good ways to help your children love their own *better than good* hair.

EDUCATION. Teach them about the dangers of using chemicals (the harmful effects on the hair, the sometimes irreversible damage to hair follicles and the scalp).

CELEBRATE NATURAL HAIR. Show your daughter pictures of gorgeous women with natural hair styled in lots of different and beautiful ways, from straight dos to afros and everything in between. They need to see positive images of women with hair like them!

PRACTICE. Lovingly care for your daughter's hair and teach her how to care for it herself. The act of caring for something and taking responsibility for it will make her appreciate it more.

SHOP. Help her get excited about natural hair care by allowing her to go shopping with you for tools and products. Let her pick out new conditioners, shampoo, and so on. Encourage a little product junkieism on her part.

MAKE HAIR TIME "US" TIME. If your daughter is old enough to ask you about relaxers, she's old enough to participate in a hair spa day with you. Put your hair spa day on the calendar and emphasize the fact that this is the day you will be spending quality time together. She'll always have fond memories of bonding with you while you did your hair. If you have more than one daughter and someone can watch the other kid(s), consider giving them each a hair session with you. They'll love the one-on-one attention.

YOUR CHILD'S HAIR ROUTINE

Remember that children are different from adults. While some of us are more than willing to drop everything and try out a new style, most children won't be. This is why it's important to focus more on establishing *a consistent hair routine* than on the hair itself. The earlier you do this, the better. If your child knows that hair time is always at such and such time, then eventually she'll come around. It's a bit like brushing their teeth. At first, most kids don't like it, but if you do it long enough, they eventually stop fighting you about it and come to accept it as a normal part of their routine. So even if you don't

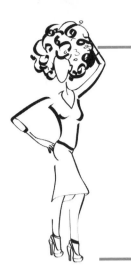

Your Mom Curlfriend Says . . .

When dealing with baby hair or children with fine hair, try leaving the conditioner in. Your daughter will enjoy smoother hair, improved curl definition, and better moisture retention.

follow our suggested routine, make sure that your hair routine is consistent if you want your child to cooperate.

WASH HAIR (ONCE A WEEK). Pick a day and always wash your child's hair on that day. It's good to pick a day like Saturday or Sunday when you have more energy, patience, and time. Make a big deal out of the fact that it's hair wash day and act really excited before you begin, like it's the equivalent of going to Disneyland.

Wash your child's hair in the bath until she's old enough to stand at the sink. Use a gentle no-tears shampoo or simply co-wash her hair with conditioner. If she's sensitive to water in her eyes, get a visor to divert the water or practice tilting her head back with her before she gets in the bathtub. (By the age of two, pointing up and telling her to "look at the ceiling" should do the trick.) Whether you choose to co-wash or shampoo, finish off with one more condition and rinse. And also be sure to seal in all that conditioning goodness with an oil or a butter.

WHILE YOUR CHILD IS STILL IN THE BATH, PUT HER HAIR INTO A PROTECTIVE STYLE like two-strand twists, bantu knots, or braids, which will get her hair nice and stretched for tomorrow morning's style.

FOR NIGHTTIME SLEEP, HAVE YOUR CHILD WEAR A SATIN CAP. If she's unwilling to keep one on, get a satin pillowcase. Those animal pillows are cute, but they can be brutal on hair. If she's old enough to be reasoned with, explain to her that she either has to accept the satin sleep cap or lose the Pillow Pet.

HAVE ALL YOUR TOOLS AT HAND THE NEXT DAY. Make sure to have everything set up before you sit your child down in the chair. You'll only try her patience if you have to keep on stopping to get some tool you're missing. Until your child is fully acclimated to her hair routine, stick to simple styles that you can do quickly and efficiently. Flat-strand twists, French braids, and simple puffs are a few of our favorite styles for children. But if you're going to try your hand at braiding, make it box braids!

Box Braids

STEP 1 On clean, damp, detangled hair, create four large sections (two in the front and two in the back).

STEP 2 Pin three sections up and out of the way.

STEP 3 Apply your moisturizer and styler of choice to the loose section of hair.

STEP 4 Section off a smaller piece of the loose section and divide it into three pieces: left, middle, and right.

STEP 5 To begin the braid, start at the roots and take the left piece and place it over the middle so that the middle piece is on the left. Then bring the right piece over to the middle.

STEP 6 Repeat Step 5 until you reach the ends of the hair. Add moisturizer or other hair product to the ends and finger curl to keep the braid from unraveling.

STEP 7 Repeat Steps 5 and 6 with the rest of that section and then do the same thing with the other three larger sections. Remember to be mindful of the edges and to keep the braids loose so that you don't create unnecessary tension at the hairline. Continuously pulling the hair too taut can result in long-term damage. Receding hairlines aren't cute on anyone, especially not your five-year-old. Sacrifice a little neatness for long-term hair and scalp health.

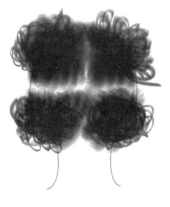

{See Step 1}

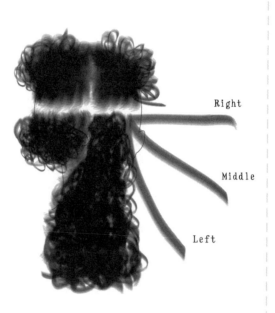

Right

Middle

Left

{See Step 4}

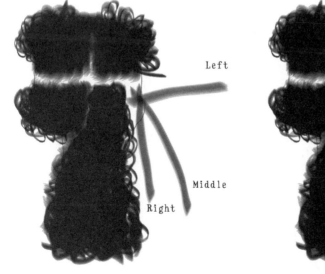

Left

Middle

Right

{See Step 5}

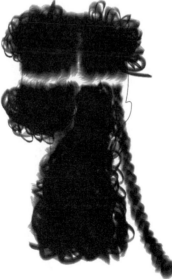

{See Step 6}

Two-Strand Twists

Instructions provided by Angela Pierre from the blog WiseCurls.com

Two-strand twists are a staple style for many moms with curly-haired kids. It provides flexibility while keeping the hair moisturized and protected. Not to mention, it allows for easy school mornings. Here's how to achieve the look recommended by curly moms everywhere.

What you'll need:

Rat tail or fine tooth comb for sectioning

Wide tooth comb for detangling

Elastic bands to hold sections in place

Moisturizer of choice for twisting

Spray bottle with your choice of oils mixed with water to keep hair moisturized during the twisting process

STEP 1 After shampooing, conditioning, and detangling hair, section it into three parts using the elastic bands. Depending on how you prefer the twists to frame your child's face, make one section of hair larger than the other two sections.

STEP 2 Start with the section of hair in the back. With your rat tail comb, part the hair from ear to ear to prepare for twisting.

STEP 3 Next, make a 1- to 1½-inch part with your rat tail comb to make your first twist. Parting allows the twists to look more uniform and neat. After you've parted the

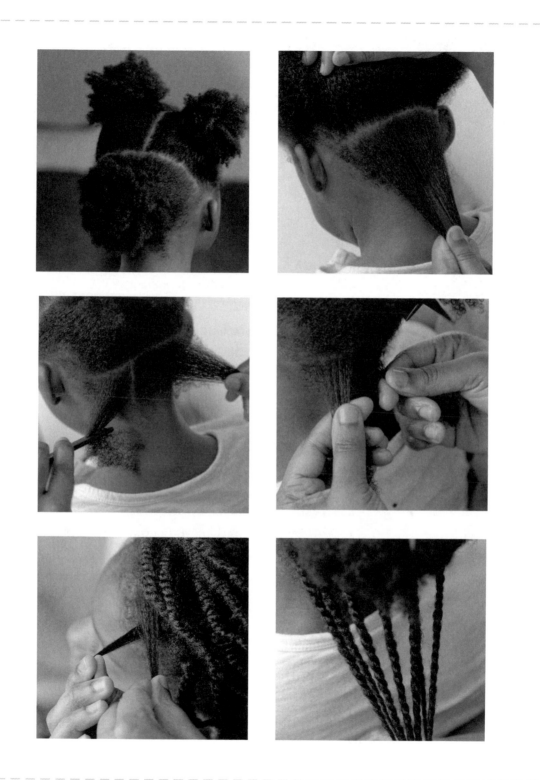

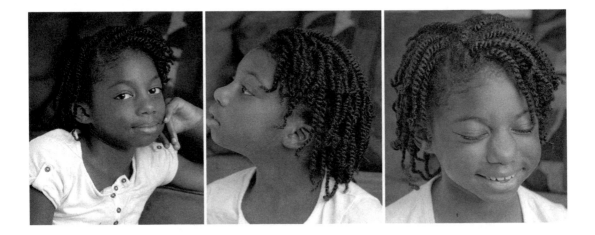

hair, take a dab of moisturizer and apply it from the roots to the ends of the hair.

STEP 4 Now that the hair is moisturized, you're ready to twist. First, split the 1- to 1½-inch section of hair into two so that you now have a smaller piece of hair between your left and right index fingers and thumbs.

In a crisscross motion, bring the left piece of hair directly over the right piece of hair. Make sure that the roots of the hair are not being pulled too tightly. Continue this motion, while stretching the hair downward, until you reach the end of the strand.

STEP 5 Repeat Steps 3 and 4. Continue this process within each section until you are complete. If the hair begins to lose moisture, give the section you're about to work on a spritz with the oil-water mixture. Allow the twists to frame your daughter's face in a way that suits her perfectly.

Cornrows

Cornrows are actually one of the simpler braiding styles, and they're a great way to practice your hair parting skills. Following are instructions for simple back-to-front cornrows, but feel free to play around with this style, especially with the part lines, which can be curved or made to go in different directions at different points of the head. Once you've conquered the simple back-to-front cornrows, you have the skills needed to do the more complicated designs.

STEP 1 Prepare your child's hair by spraying it with either water or a leave-in conditioner. With the tail of your rat tail comb, make a part down the middle of your child's head, from the forehead to the nape. Parting will take practice.

STEP 2 Clip or tie off the hair on the left side. You'll be working with the hair on the right first.

STEP 3 Decide how many rows you want on each side. For the purpose of these instructions, we'll go with three rows on each side, but depending on your child's hair length (and patience), you'll be able to do a minimum of two rows to a side or—if *you* have the patience—several small ones.

STEP 4 Part a third of the hair closest to the ear and clip back the rest of the section. This part may be a little more curved to accommodate the ear line, but try to make the part as clean as possible.

STEP 5 Work a water-based moisturizer through the section you are about to braid, then seal it in with an oil.

Depending on your child's hair texture, you may opt to use a styler for an extra bit of hold.

STEP 6 Take a small section at the front of the section you'll be braiding and split it into three equal pieces. Start with the hair on the right and cross it under the middle piece. Then take the piece on the left and cross that under the middle piece.

STEP 7 On the next pass, gather some hair from the unbraided section into the piece on the far right, then pass this new piece under the middle. The hair gathered into the braid should be about equal in size to the pieces you began with when you first started braiding.

STEP 8 Take the left piece, gather some loose hair into it, and cross it under the middle.

STEP 9 Repeat Steps 7 and 8 until you reach the nape. Watch out for stray hairs and smooth them into the cornrows as you go along. The key to terrific cornrows is clean parts and keeping them neat as you braid.

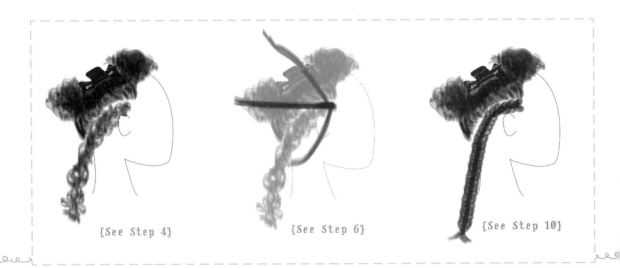

{See Step 4}   {See Step 6}   {See Step 10}

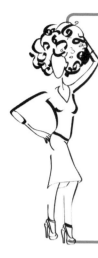

STEP 10 When you reach the nape, braid the rest of the hair as you would a regular braid. You can braid all the way to the end, or for easier take down, stop about an inch from the end, divide the remaining loose hair into two sections, and twist to the end. In either case, use a pomade to seal the tips.

STEP 11 Repeat Steps 5 through 10 on the rest of the head.

WHEN YOUR CHILD'S HAIR ISN'T LIKE YOUR OWN

We consider ourselves lucky to be living in a gorgeous world, where all sorts of family structures can come together. There are more multiracial kids than ever before in the United States. And more and more couples are completing their families with the adoption of black children.

The White Mother of a Beautiful, Brilliant Toddler

By Karen Valby

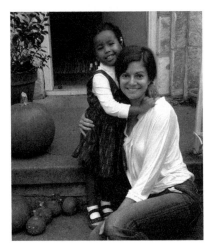

White women love to sigh over my daughter Ava's hair and the efforts I must put into it. "I bet that took a long time," they say. It did take a long time, I want to tell them. I'm the white mother of a beautiful, brilliant three-and-a-half-year-old black girl.

When we met she was eleven months old, and I didn't know how to tell a good conditioner from a bad one. I didn't know where to find a sleep cap for toddlers or when to use a brush or a comb or my fingers. I bought and threw out a lot of products. I redid a lot of parts. I watched a lot of YouTube videos. I asked some dumb questions. I got pretty good at twists. My cornrows are a work in progress. But I put in the time, which in my book equals love, because one of my jobs in this world is to be worthy of my child's hair.

When my daughter turned three, I realized that I'd become shamefully reliant on puffs, and I was noticing some breakage around her hairline. It was time for my repertoire to grow. So I ordered some beads and a threader and clasps. I gave her too many snacks and let her gorge on starch and TV, so I could do her hair in peace. And I'm telling you, my first attempt at box braids was a thing of beauty. The parts were clean; the design of them somehow seemed predetermined rather than a lucky accident. I wanted to cry at the end, not just because I was proud of my efforts but because my child no longer looked like a baby. And because when I sent her off to look at herself in the mirror, she marveled at her reflection. All of us should know what it feels like to stare back at ourselves with such pride and admiration.

That afternoon we went to the home of a white girlfriend for a playdate. At one point Ava called out to the room of children, "Whoever has braids in their hair gets to be the leader!"

Meanwhile her girlfriend, a peach of a thing with extremely fine blond hair, looked longingly at Ava's braids, coveting her pink and purple and clear iridescent beads that clacked happily when she jumped and ran. Her friend tugged on my arm later as we were saying good-bye.

"Do you think you could make my hair look like Ava's sometime?" she wondered hopefully. I picked up the ends of her lank hair, pinching the entire slip of it between my thumb and forefinger. *Oh dear*, I thought. It would take some time, but I could try.

Karen Valby is a senior writer at *Entertainment Weekly*. Her nonfiction book *Welcome to Utopia: Notes from a Small Town* is now out in paperback. She lives in Austin, Texas, with her family and spends her Sunday afternoons doing hair.

However, when it comes to the differences in hair texture, it isn't always kumbaya. We receive hundreds of notes every year from mothers and fathers of black and multiracial children that basically boil down to "How do I do this child's hair?" Here are some tips for achieving better than good hair for your children, even if their hair isn't like your own.

1. KNOW THAT BLACK WOMEN AREN'T BORN KNOWING HOW TO DO THEIR CHILD'S HAIR. There's a reason that

kids are getting relaxers at younger ages. Even if you're not the same race or gender as your children, you may be working with the exact same skill set as a black mother who doesn't already have natural hair. Don't assume that your race, gender, or history puts you at a disadvantage for doing your child's hair. Just commit to learning how to do her or his type of hair. And most of all, be patient with yourself. It's okay to make mistakes on the road to the perfect protective style. Give yourself at least a year to learn your child's hair, and don't go into it with a defeatist attitude. Doing your child's hair is not rocket science.

2. REACH OUT! REACH OUT! REACH OUT! WE'LL BE THERE. A lot of nonblack mothers tell us that they feel too intimidated to do exactly what we do, which is *ask other black women for hair advice.* Don't worry about offending your fellow mom at the PTA or the woman in line in the grocery store. Ask for help! Nine times out of ten, they will want you to ask them, especially if your child's hair is a mess. You're more likely to find yourself on the unexpected end of a barrage of advice, rather than having offended the person you asked. So when you see a child whose hair looks the way you want your child's hair to look, simply compliment the child's mother and pick her brain for how she achieved that look. She'll probably be more than happy to share.

3. EXPERIMENT. Listen, not every parent—black or of any other ethnicity—is meant for box braiding.

This is no reflection on you or your parenting skills. Simply experiment with different styles until you find the perfect fit. Engineering type? Try a style that requires precise parting. Got smaller fingers? You might be a whiz at bantu knots. Crunchy granola? You could definitely have what it takes to conquer the all-natural afro. Remember that you'll never know which styles you'll be good or great at until you try a lot of them. And keep on trying. One of the best ways to help your child love her or his own hair is to take an active, fun, and loving interest in it.

No matter what your ethnicity, gender, or current skill level, if you practice, experiment, and seek out advice, your kid's hair is going to look fabulous. Just be forewarned: it's going to make running errands a bit harder when everyone's stopping you to compliment you on your kid's hair! Many of our curlfriends have found this out the hard way.

BOYS, BOYS, BOYS

As we said earlier in this chapter, a lot of moms take their boys to get their hair lopped off as soon as they can sit up in a barber chair. And there really is nothing wrong with that, especially if you're short on time as many mothers are. But do keep in mind that even though boys' hair requires much less maintenance than girls' hair, it's not absolutely *no-*

A Special Note to the Parents of Multiracial Children

By Ernessa T. Carter

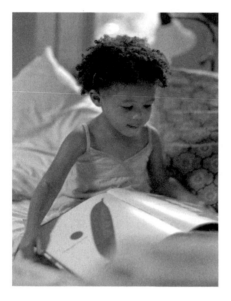

It's been an amazing and eye-opening experience coauthoring a book about natural hair. When Nikki and I first started out, we thought it would be a fairly straightforward thing, but it turned out to be so much more than that. I can still remember sending her an e-mail after we finished the rough draft that basically said, "Whew, it feels like we just took a *journey*."

But I think the most important lesson that I've taken away from this book is not to compare hair. It's easy to forget that not all biracial children have "the same kind of hair," even the ones who like my daughter have a black mother and a white father. What works for your biracial daughter might not work for mine. And while I've been lucky to receive so much advice from biracial women and other mothers of biracial children, to my surprise, the biggest breakthrough came from Roberta Valderrama, a wonderfully fierce and curly Peruvian American actress who told me at a mutual friend's baby shower to condition my daughter's hair with Aussie Moist and just leave it in. My biggest piece of advice to you is to stay open to advice from others. Receive it with gratitude from *everyone*: black mothers, nonblack curlies, hairdressers—everyone has wisdom to share.

My other piece of advice is to experiment. Don't settle on any one product. Though I swear by Mixed Chicks Leave-in Conditioner and argan oil for my own daughter's hair, I'm continuously switching things out, just to see how something new will work. I recently found out that the cornrows and flat-strand twists I put in my daughter's hair on Monday mornings will last for a whole forty-eight hours if I seal in the Mixed Chicks Leave-in Conditioner with Carol's Daughters Mimosa Hair Honey. Also, trial and error has taught me that while I can go two weeks between washes, my daughter can only go one. And while I'd love to use a fancier shampoo or just do a co-wash on her hair, if I want to have a cooperative toddler, I had best use tear-free shampoo and call it a day.

You can't learn everything from reading a book; you'll have to experiment on your own. But the natural hair routine we posted earlier in this chapter is a great jumping-off point until you figure out what's best for your multiracial child's hair.

Just remember the following tips:

BIRTH TO ONE YEAR

KEEP THE ROUTINE VERY SIMPLE. Just co-wash with a tear-free conditioner, use Aussie Moist or a leave-in conditioner, and seal in the moisture with baby oil.

TODDLERS

WASH YOUR CHILD'S HAIR ONCE A WEEK. Co-washing is great if you can find a conditioner that does the job and doesn't burn your child's eyes if she refuses to wear a water visor or tilt her head back. Otherwise, try washing with a tear-free shampoo and then use a leave-in conditioner like Mixed Chicks or Aussie Moist if you don't want to buy a more expensive one.

PUT YOUR CHILD'S HAIR IN A PROTECTIVE STYLE AT NIGHT. Think of stretching styles such as bantu knots, two-strand twists, or loose braids. The most important thing is to create a protective style around what you want her hair to look like the next morning. For example, if you want her to wear her hair loose with a side part the next morning, make the side part first, then put her hair in a protective style. If you want to put her in a headband with bangs, separate the bangs from the rest of the hair and style them in the direction you want them to hang. If you simply want to stretch her hair or maintain curl definition, then you can pretty much do whatever you want.

STYLE YOUR CHILD'S HAIR IN THE MORNING. More intricate styles like cornrows, French braids, and flat twists are better done in the morning—especially if your toddler refuses to wear a sleep cap. Otherwise, you can undo her nighttime protective style and either let her wear it out or restyle it into something more durable, like puffs.

maintenance. In fact, their hair and scalp will thrive if you stick to these simple rules.

Every Three Months

CUT OR TRIM OR DUST. Even if you're going for length, boys still need the occasional trim or dust to manage split ends. For more on DIY dusting, see our dusting instructions in chapter 4.

Every Week

WASH OR CO-WASH ONCE A WEEK. If you want to go a step above Johnson & Johnson, try a nonfragrant or nonflowery shampoo such as Matrix Biolage Shampoo, Elucence Moisture Benefits Shampoo, or Giovanni 50:50 Balanced Hydrating-Clarifying Shampoo followed by either an instant conditioner like Aveda Be Curly Conditioner, Aussie Moist, or Curls Coconut Sublime Conditioner and, last but not least, a leave-in such as Paul Mitchell The Conditioner, SheaMoisture Coconut and Hibiscus Conditioning Milk, or Curls Milkshake. The good news is that if you leave your son's hair short, washing won't take long at all.

PUT IT IN A PROTECTIVE STYLE IF YOU'RE GOING FOR LENGTH. Cornrows (see page 155) have been the go-to style of generations, and this is the perfect way for your son to get both his play and his grow on. Don't worry if yours leave a lot to be desired at first; just keep on practicing and refer to our "Hair Squirm Busters" on page 141 if your son doesn't cooperate.

Every Day

IN THE MORNING, spritz your son's hair with water, then either put in a nonfragrant leave-in like Qhemet Biologics Cocoa Tree Detangling Ghee or use a spritz leave-in that works for both sexes, such as Oyin Handmade's Greg Juice or Frank Juice, then seal in the moisture with an unscented oil such as jojoba. If you're getting close to the time when you'll need to take him to the barber, rub a little leave-in or styling pomade into your hands and individually tweak each runaway curl so that it will look neater.

If you're going for length and want your son to wear his hair out, undo his protective style, spritz it with water, use either a cream or a spritz leave-in (his hair will let you know which one it prefers), then rub your hands with an unscented oil like glycerin and use your fingers to "comb" it out and shape it into an afro or, in the case of some biracial curlies, a style that hangs.

For either short or long hair, be prepared to use a pomade to lay down the edges.

AT NIGHT, put the hair in a protective style if you're going for length, even if you want your son to wear his hair out every day. It doesn't need to be neat or even formally parted. Sloppy cornrows or something as simple as two braids will do.

I've Got Two Boy Children

By Jamyla Bennu of Oyin Handmade

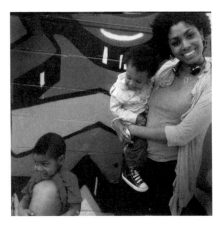

I come from a family where no one cuts Baby's hair before his second birthday. I also come from a gene pool where babies tend to be born with heads full of thick hair, so I have ushered my two boy children from firstborn wispiness through their transitional baby curls and coils and onward to their fully realized textures. Now I have lots of experience with texture and hair care.

With each of our sons, we have used the principles of gentle, moisturizing hair care from the start. Having good care practices along with easy care styles (and a somewhat forgiving attitude about final presentation) helps us to keep their care needs to a minimum while instilling good hair health routines into their lives. We think that the following tips are a good start whether a child's hair is kept short or encouraged to grow long.

* **CLEANSE GENTLY.** We wash our sons' hair with a moisturizing castile-based gentle cleanser. (We use Oyin's Honey Wash from head to toe.)
* **CONDITION OFTEN.** We do conditioner rinses in between cleansings when their scalps are clean but the hair needs some refreshing.
* **DETANGLE GENTLY.** We detangle hair while it is wet and soaked in conditioner, using our fingers or a soft shower brush.
* **MOISTURIZE WELL.** After we wash their hair, we leave a touch of

conditioner in to help retain moisture, or we apply a liquid leave-in spray (glycerin-rich to help the hair retain and draw moisture) or a creamy leave-in hair lotion. Either of these products is applied while the hair is wet.

* **DRY GENTLY.** We let their coils air-dry overnight.
* **STYLE GENTLY.** In the mornings, we do a quick spritz with water or one of the Oyin juices and then either fluff or mold their hair into shape for the day.

Currently, the boys are one and four. "The prequel" sports a *Kirikou-and-the-Sorceress*-inspired half mohawk, which rises to a triangular pyramid of pen-spring-size coils in the front and tapers to a close-cropped point in the middle of his crown. My husband cuts our son's hair about once or twice a month, usually while his current favorite attention-holding movie is playing to help mitigate the squirms and protests.

"The sequel" still has his never-been-cut baby fluff, which looks perpetually as though he has stuck his finger in a light socket. To style his wild tufty fro, we just spritz with water or Oyin juices every day or two, and massage.

I will admit that although I mourn my lack of girls when it comes time for clothes shopping, I do sometimes feel like I got off easy in the hair care department, what with the cultural acceptability of shaving my children's heads and all. But that doesn't mean I got off altogether.

- -

Jamyla Bennu is the creative visionary behind Oyin Handmade—a naturally nourishing, affordable, luxurious line of handmade hair and skin care products. Self-described as "crafty, nerdy, and fun-loving," the modern-day Renaissance woman juggles her numerous responsibilities as mixtress, entrepreneur, wife, business partner, and mother of two small boys. Jamyla and her husband, artist and filmmaker Pierre Bennu, were named the Coolest Black Family in America in the first feature of an ongoing series by Ebony.com.

MOTHERING WHILE CURLY

Nikki says: I peer off into the not-so-distant past occasionally and see a time in my life when the only thing I was genuinely concerned about was whether my henna would arrive prior to Saturday, or, as I referred to it back then, "spa day." During this period in my life, before child (BC), I styled two, sometimes three times a week. I frequently tried new hairstyles and new products, and I spent much of my time on the Web chatting it up with other curlfriends. BC, I could go to work, come home, and spontaneously decide to see a movie with the hubs, or head out for drinks at our favorite bar. On the weekends, you could find me with my curlfriends at the lounge, swinging our fros and living it up. It was a beautiful time, a good time, but as most good things do, it came to an end.

Things are different now. Not bad, just different. When my beautiful daughter, Gia (aka Boogie), made her grand entrance into the world, everything pretty much halted. My fast-paced life has become more of a crawl, and me time has become, sadly, nonexistent. I've been busted down to one, maybe two, tried-and-true, go-to hairstyles. And spa day? A mere memory. Heck, I barely have time to shower.

In the beginning, I must admit that things were much more difficult than they are now, because back then everything was so new, and it took a lot of getting used to. More than a year in now, we've snuggled into a comfortable routine, and I'm back to washing my hair at least twice a month! So that's good.

It is definitely a balancing act, and if nothing else, becoming a mother has helped me put some things into perspective. I'm a notoriously anal person: I'm very punctual and very organized, and I live and die by my thoughtfully composed to-do list. When I couldn't do something I needed (or rather wanted) to do "right now," I used to freak out. Well, Gia's learned me. *My* schedule no longer exists. I'm doing what I can around nap time, playtime, Boogie time, and so on, and it's been good for me.

Learning to go with the flow and relinquish control wasn't in *The Mocha Manual to a Fabulous Pregnancy* (neither was dealing with liquid poop). My advice for the other natural child-work-hubby-hair-juggling divas out there is to keep your heads up. Take care of the family, but don't forget about yourself. In order to be the best mom you can be, you have to be happy with yourself. If that means asking someone else to step in and take the little one somewhere while you sneak in a henna session (or a secret nap), so be it. A happy, healthy, beautified you will be much more capable of dealing with the occasional diaper blowout. Trust me.

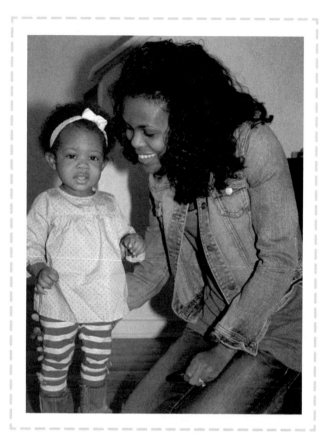

NATURAL KIDS AND MOMS SOUND OFF!

I think my daughter's hair texture will be fine like mine. Because of what I've been learning about my own natural hair over the last couple of years, I feel much more confident about combing and caring for her hair. I'm not intimidated by it all, and I look forward to getting to know her hair in the way that I'm learning about mine.

I expect to teach her (and my husband, because it's important for him too!) how to:

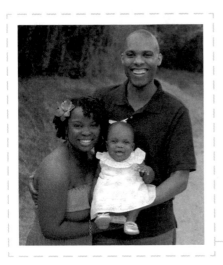

* ***Care for her hair*** *by keeping it clean, handling it gently, and protecting it.*

* ***Embrace her hair*** *and know that every day won't be a fabulous hair day! Your curls will defy and frustrate you. Yet and still, you have to just roll with it and make it work!*

* ***Love her hair.*** *The key here is that your hair is a part of you, just like your face, hands, and feet. You have to love and be confident in your whole self and not be defined by any one part.*

—Amber Wright (pictured with her husband and daughter)

Tip 1: No towel drying your curls. This simple step has changed the natural hair game for me and Chloe. We have "borrowed" a bunch of her dad's white undershirts! On a wash-and-go for Chloe (because she has mad length and volume), we do the plopping method, which absorbs the excess water and product while clumping her curls. When we let her hair down, it is so beautiful! For other styles we use the neck of the undershirt to frame her head and hairline and twist the end like a turban to soak up the water until I'm ready to do her hair.

Tip 2: Use water and your five fingers for detangling. With my spray bottle filled with good ol' H_2O, finger detangling is a breeze. If there are any pesky curly knots, we apply conditioner and they come right out.

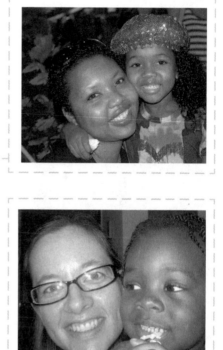

Tip 3: Pre-poo with oil. I use extra virgin olive oil and twist Chloe's hair in six to eight sections, put a satin bonnet on her, and call it a night. Her hair is supermoisturized, and after I wash it, it feels so soft.

—Michelle Parker (pictured with Chloe)

Being an adoptive mom, I've had to learn all about my little one's hair as she grows. We tell her how fun her curls are and how beautiful she is. She loves to play with her hair and now is trying to play with mine. She is noticing the difference between her hair and mine and many of her friends' hair, too. So far she likes to get her hair done and loves when I leave it out, too.

—Lesa E (pictured with Marlee E)

When it comes to taking care of my daughter's hair, it helps a ton that I went natural! She's only two years old, but she knows that our hair is the same. She'll like a style I have in my hair, and she'll say, "Mommy, my hairs too!" She's already rocking twist-outs, braid-outs, and the ever infamous satin bonnet at night! At her age, it's monkey see, monkey do. So when it's Mommy's hair "spa" day, it's hers, too. She knows she's naturally beautiful because I tell

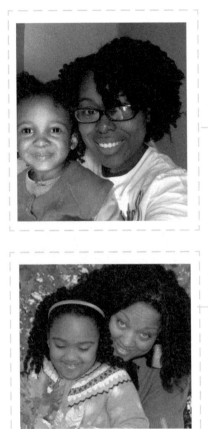

her all the time. I'm sure I'm already raising a mini product junkie. She gets excited whenever I buy hair products for myself and says, "Mine? For my hairs pretty?" and I gently say, "No, not yours . . . ours."

—Tenesha Bailey (pictured with Aubrey)

My daughter is one of the reasons I went natural. She is seven years old, and I have been natural for about three years. Early on, I always told her how beautiful her hair was and how important it is to take care of it. Now that she is older, she continues to love her curls and looks forward to when we take twists out to see how curly they are!

—Ylandus Roundy (pictured with M. Symone)

CHAPTER SIX

All Grown Up Now

Dealing With Long Hair

Hair, glorious hair! Perhaps one doesn't truly understand the lyrics to the musical *Hair*'s eponymous song until the main character reaches the much longed-for stage of having long tresses. At this stage, you gain the emotional satisfaction of having finally reached your goal as well as the ability to achieve just about any hairstyle you come across, from defined waves to striking updos. And the compliments—don't even get us started on the compliments. At this point you might actually have become sick and tired of everybody and their mama stopping you in the grocery store to tell you how much they love your hair

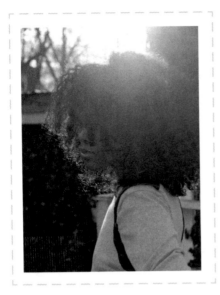

(but not really—hair compliments are always in fashion).

However, just like every other stage of your natural journey, this one comes with its share of trials and tribulations. It's ironic, because you've been working all these years to achieve long, healthy hair, and when you finally do, you realize that this means you've actually got to deal with having a lot of hair. Here are the top five issues our curlfriends with longer hair have reported to us.

THE FIVE BIGGEST LONG HAIR ISSUES

1. LONGER AND MORE FRUSTRATING DETANGLING SESSIONS. Once your hair goes beyond your bra strap, expect detangling sessions to last in excess of forty-five minutes. Music star Corinne Bailey Rae says it takes her nearly an hour to detangle her gorgeous head of hair, so she does it in her garden to at least make it scenic and interesting. See page 177 for other suggestions on what to do while doing your hair.

2. DEALING WITH OLDER ENDS THAT NEED TLC. Even if you're as gentle as you can possibly be with your ends—which most of us aren't—they can still become weak and prone to splits, knots, and

THINGS TO DO WHILE DOING YOUR DO

Most of us tend to watch our favorite TV shows or a movie during longer hair sessions. But what happens when your DVR list is empty and there's no movie or show you particularly want to see? Here are some suggestions:

* Listen in full to that new album you downloaded. Get out of your musical rut while you put in a fabulous style.

* No time to read? Listen to an audiobook while tackling your hair.

* If you're in college, this is a great time to study notes or run flash cards with a curlfriend.

* One curlfriend told us she's been teaching herself Spanish, so she watches movies in Spanish while she does her hair. *¡Muy bueno!*

* Throw a curl party. Invite some curlfriends over to do hair and have cocktails. This is even better than a girls' night out.

* Book club your hair. You can get your hair done and discuss the book your book club just finished. How's that for *well*-read?

* Another one for the college curlies: Get together for a curlfriend chat and style party. You can discuss all manner of topics while getting your style on.

* Listen to a comedy album. Old Paul Mooney stand-up shows are a personal favorite of Nikki's.

* Use your hands-free earbuds or Bluetooth to catch up with a friend while putting in your twists.

* Start thinking about your next style by watching YouTube natural hair tutorials while you put in the current one.

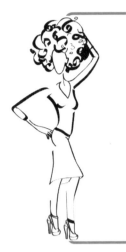

breakage. Regular trimming becomes even more of a necessity with longer hair.

3. LONGER STYLING TIME. Twisting short hair can take up to thirty minutes, so imagine how long it takes to do a twist-out on longer hair! If you want the defined curls you see in the magazines and online, you'll have to put in the time to get them.

4. SAYING GOOD-BYE TO A FEW OF YOUR STANDBY STYLES. You don't really know how much you love a puff until your ability to wear your hair in one is gone. And wash-and-gos at this stage can leave you with knots galore. In general, it's not a great idea to wash-and-go with longer hair, as the tangling and matting can make for a miserable wash day.

5. EXPENSIVE OR MO' HAIR, MO' PRODUCTS. Having lots of hair requires more products to keep it healthy and looking good. Nikki goes through a shocking amount of conditioner every month, and if your hair is addicted to a product that isn't cheap, the costs can

SCARVES ARE A CURL'S BEST FRIEND!

Instructions provided by Shanti Mayers

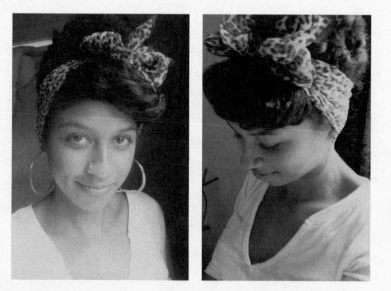

To get the look shown in the pictures here, do the following:

* This look is best with hair that has texture to it, so do this on a fresh twist-out or recently unbraided hair.

* Take a section from the front of your hair and cross it to the opposite side creating a side bang. Secure it with bobby pins.

* Gently roll the remaining hair into a French twist and secure it with bobby pins. If desired, create the French twist with emphasis on the top to give the look height and volume (as pictured).

* Wrap a small scarf around your head (hiding the bobby pins) so that the ends meet at the top of your head, and tie it into a cute bow.

really add up! Here are a few tips for maintaining long hair without emptying out your wallet.

* USE WHAT YOU ALREADY HAVE. Don't keep running out and buying the next best thing. Now is the time to put yourself in product junkie rehab.

* USE LESS PRODUCT. Don't be so heavy-handed. Oftentimes with hair, less is more. Product buildup can lead to problems down the road. Plus, it's difficult to achieve big, fluffy hair with heavy locks weighed down with product. Your products will go further if you use less of them and add more only if needed. Start with a little and add more slowly.

* APPLY PRODUCT IN SECTIONS. You'll often use less when you do this, and it gets distributed more evenly.

* TAKE YOUR HAIR GAME TO THE NEXT LEVEL AND MAKE YOUR OWN PRODUCTS. You can make your own deep conditioners (see our recipe in chapter 2, on page 54), pre-poos (a mix of oils

Your Best Curlfriend Says . . .

Feel free to go cheap on the conditioners you use for detangling. Products such as Herbal Essences Hello Hydration provide great slippage without leaving a hole in your wallet.

and conditioner), and leave-in conditioning spritzes (oil, water, and veggie glycerin). Homemade spritzes and butters are very popular on hair message boards, and they can be incredibly beneficial. If you decide to become your own mixtress, please make sure you're adding preservatives to your concoctions and/or keeping them refrigerated.

* ADD OILS AND OTHER INGREDIENTS TO YOUR CONDITIONERS TO HELP THEM STRETCH. But remember that products can spoil when you introduce water and oils to them. We suggest pouring some of your favorite conditioner into a smaller bottle and adding your oils and water to that to thin out the product. Dispose of or refrigerate what you don't use.

* MASTER SECOND- AND THIRD-DAY HAIR. Get a nighttime routine and stick to it! If you're only doing your hair once or twice a week, you'll use less product.

* ROCK MORE UPDOS. Go back to chapter 4 and learn how to turn limp frizzy curls into cute updos so that you can make your wash day efforts last longer.

* * *

While having long hair comes with its share of issues, most of our curlfriends report great satisfaction with their long hair. No, you can't do wash-and-gos anymore or thirty-minute twist-outs, but you can throw your hair into a couple of super-quick sloppy braids at night and still come out looking fabulous the next morning. Also, if you don't feel like dealing with your hair, you don't have to. You can simply put it in a bun or a ponytail when you're frustrated with it or need it out of your way. It's also easier both to keep long hair out of your face when you work out and to get gorgeous second- and third-day hair.

When you achieve a head of long, healthy hair, you've made it to the highest point in your natural hair journey. You've educated yourself, you've experimented, and now you've developed a truly amazing relationship with your hair. Congratulations!

In the coming years, keep in mind that your hair will continue to transform. Our curlfriends have reported changes in texture, porosity, and color due to factors such as age, pregnancy, or even just moving to an area with a different climate. So even if you think you know your hair now, keep in mind that it can and probably will change in several ways over the next few years. Stay open to experimentation and innovation, and please use this book as a touchstone for every surprise your hair throws at you.

You'll never stop having a relationship with your hair, and we wish you a continued journey rich in surprises, learning, and love.

EPILOGUE

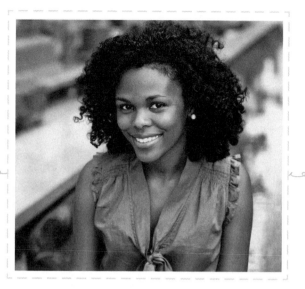

You're still here? Great! I was hoping we didn't lose you. I'm sure at times you may have become a little overwhelmed. Like, "Does it really take all of this?!" But we had to lay it out there like that. Trust me, it's not as hard as it looks at first read, and it most certainly gets easier with time and practice. *(Ahem.)* Well, that's not entirely true, seeing as how time brings about change. And at different lengths, in different environments, under different conditions, and with different products, our hair can behave like some wicked little child you've never before seen.

But know this: learning about your natural hair, caring for it, styling it, and experimenting with it is never in vain. Yes, there will be times that you want to rip it out and trade it in for someone else's, and some days, you'll want to shave it all off and start over. But nothing worth having is easy to achieve, and a head full of healthy, natural hair is no different.

I've been in this game for years now. I've done it all and tried it all, and I've made it into a lifestyle that has transcended my natural hair and become a part of who I am. Going natural is about more than just "not using relaxers." If that was all this was about, there would be no natural hair movement, no books, no websites, and no meet-ups. I've talked to countless natural celebs and hundreds, maybe thousands, of natural hair women, and through my interactions with them I have concluded that your typical curlfriend:

* Loves to look and feel good. This is why every girl she meets admires her confidence, and every dude she meets admires her confidence, among other things.
* Is never without her satin cap or satin-covered pillow.
* Hates to be put in a box. *(Don't stereotype me, boo-boo!)*
* Doesn't run from the rain—unless she's rocking a wicked twist-out!
* Loves to change it up every now and then and flat-iron her hair but within a week is ready to wash and resurrect her curls.
* Never questions whether her hair is professional enough or appropriate enough for some event or gala.
* Always takes her vitamins.
* Doesn't want her hair to be petted. *(No, it doesn't have a name. No, you can't take it home.)*
* Eats healthy but allows for the occasional splurge. She's very mindful of what she puts on and in her body.
* Doesn't settle.
* Loves to water her hair and body.
* Is effortlessly chic and fashionable.
* Walks down the street like a model.
* Struts into a room and immediately owns it.

* Can talk hair for hours and hours.
* Has never met a "curly stranger." Two curlfriends meeting for the first time = Celie and Nettie reuniting. (Clasps hands and sings ♪♪♪ "You and I must neeever paaart." ♪♪♪)
* Watches reruns of *GirlFriends* to gawk at Tracee Ellis Ross's hair.
* Is a true mixtress and can make a conditioner out of kitchen ingredients. She is to her hair what Rachael Ray is to a soufflé.
* Loves a new curly product.
* Lives on CurlyNikki.com.

Most of all, a true curlfriend loves herself and loves her hair!

Happy Hair Journey!

Nikki Walton

SPECIAL THANKS

The absolute best aspect of being part of the natural hair community is the willingness of all its members to both give and receive accumulated wisdom. We are especially grateful to all of the curlfriends who contributed their time, tips, essays, styling instructions, and supercute photos to this book, including:

Alexandra Smith from *The Good Hair Blog*
(http://thegoodhairblog.com/)

Amber Wright from *The YeYo Diaries*
(http://theyeyodiaries.wordpress.com/)

Angela Pierre from WiseCurls.com
(http://wisecurls.com/)

Antoinette and Shanti from *Around the Way Curls*
(http://www.acurlsbf.com/)

Charnika "CharyJay" Jett from Chary-Jay.com
(http://chary-jay.com/)

Chatel Theagene from *Back to Curly*
(http://backtocurly.com/)

Danielle Faust from *OK, Dani*
(http://okdani.com)

GG Renee Hill from *The Write Curl Diary*
(http://www.thewritecurldiary.com/)

Jamyla Bennu from Oyin Handmade
(https://www.oyinhandmade.com/)

Jonathon Anderson Pharm D of CurlyNikki.com

Leandra Williams from *What My World's Like*
(http://www.whatmyworldslike.com/blog/)

LV Burns from *Natural-ness*
(http://cbpublish.com/myhairjourney_files/)

Nadine Afia from the "GirlsLoveYourCurls" YouTube channel
(http://www.youtube.com/user/GirlsLoveYourCurls)

Nichelle Gainer from *Vintage Black Glamour*
(http://vintageblackglamour.tumblr.com/)

Nicole Harmon from *Hair Liberty*
(http://www.hairliberty.org/black-hair-care/)

Ni-Kiya Alleyne from the "Bambii by Two :)"
YouTube channel
(http://www.youtube.com/user/bambiix2/videos)

Patricia K. Perry, M.D., of DermClear, Inc.

Savvy Brown from *Savvy Brown*
(http://savvybrown.com/)

Shelli Gillis from *Hairscapades*
(http://hairscapades.com/)

Sherrell Dorsey from *Organic Beauty Vixen*
(http://www.organicbeautyvixen.com/)

Tenisha Mercer from *The Hairnista Chronicles*
(http://hairnista.blogspot.com)

TiaShauntee from *Her Best Hair*
(http://www.tiashauntee.com/)

Your Natural Hair Product Guide

Whether you're transitioning or a natural hair veteran, this product list is a great place to start. If you're trying a new hair routine, figure out what your hair needs are and choose products designed to address those needs. Try the routine for three weeks, then reassess and determine if you need to go back to the drawing board. Don't try too many new things at once, and keep a journal—documentation is often the key to great hair. Take pictures of your results as you go along and record how various product combos work for you.

Just remember, no two heads are alike, and what works for some will not work for all. Keep experimenting!

KEY

NS	Nonsulfate shampoo
🐷	Money-savers
CC	Suitable for the "conscious curly": a curly who takes care to use the most natural products she can find.
LCC	Suitable for the "loose cannon curly": a curly who uses whatever she can find as long as it's in her price range. Ingredients don't matter much to the loose cannon curly, but effectiveness does!
♡	Nikki Fave! A product that Nikki uses, loves, and highly recommends!

CLEANSERS

Pre-poos

The cleansing process, while necessary, can be stressful on our delicate strands. Shampoo can strip hair of vital oils and leave strands rough and tangled. A pre-poo is a treatment applied prior to shampooing that consists of oils and/or conditioners. It is usually performed to help the hair retain necessary moisture during the drying shampoo process. Pre-poo treatments greatly reduce hygral fatigue—the expanding and contracting of hair as water enters and exits—and help maintain the structural integrity of the cuticle and the cortex. Pre-pooing also makes hair easier to detangle, which results in less breakage when it's combed. Most moisturizing deep or instant conditioners or oils can be used to pre-poo!

BRICK AND MORTAR

Burt's Bees Avocado Butter Pre-Shampoo Hair Treatment (CC, 🐷)

Castor oil (CC, 🐷)

Extra virgin olive oil (CC, 🐷)

Grape seed oil (CC, 🐷)

Virgin coconut oil (CC, 🐷)

Vatika oil (LCC, 🐷)

ONLINE

Jessicurl Deep Conditioning Treatment (CC)

Jessicurl Too Shea! Extra Moisturizing Conditioner (CC, ♡)

Curl Junkie Rehab Moisturizing Hair Treatment (CC)

Curl Junkie Hibiscus and Banana (CC)

Myhoneychild Olive You (CC, ♡)

Shampoos

Every natural hair routine needs a good, effective shampoo. You can shampoo as often as you deem necessary. Curlies who use heavier products, stylers, and butters may shampoo as often as once a week or prior to every styling session, while the minimalists (folks who use lighter products) may shampoo once a month or biweekly. Nikki shampoos when her hair feels gunky, which is usually twice a month.

No matter how often you shampoo, moisture retention should be a top priority. Even with the milder options listed here, pre-poos (moisturizing treatments applied prior to shampooing) or deep treatments (moisturizing treatments applied following shampooing) are essential!

BRICK AND MORTAR FINDS

As I Am Cleansing Pudding (CC, NS)

Alberto VO5 Moisture Milk Moisturizing Shampoo (LCC, 🐷)

Alberto VO5 Tea Therapy Shampoo (LCC, 🐷)

Aveda BeCurly Shampoo (CC, NS)

Aveda Dry Remedy Shampoo (CC, NS)

Aveda Shampure Shampoo (CC, NS)

Aveeno Nourish and Moisturize Shampoo (CC, 🐷)

Big by Lush (CC, NS)

Cabellina For Mane, Tail & Body Shampoo (LCC, 🐷)

Carol's Daughter Rosemary Mint Clarifying Shampoo (CC, NS)

Cream of Nature Detangling Conditioner Shampoo (LCC, 🐷)

Curls Curlicious Curls Cleansing Cream (CC, NS)

Curly Wurly by Lush (CC, NS)

Cynthia Silvia Stout by Lush (CC, NS)

DevaCare No-Poo or Low-Poo (CC, NS)

DevaCurl No-Poo or Low-Poo (CC, NS)

Dove Daily Moisture Shampoo (LCC, 🐷)

Dr. Peppermint by Lush (CC, NS)

Garnier Fructis Daily Care Shampoo (LCC, 🐷)

Garnier Fructis Length and Strength Shampoo (LCC, 🐷)

Garnier Fructis Triple Nutrition Shampoo (LCC, 🐷)

Giovanni Shampoo 50:50 Balanced Hydrating-Clarifying (CC, NS, 🐷)

Giovanni Tea Tree Triple Treat Shampoo (LCC, 🐷)

Herbal Essences Hello Hydration Shampoo (LCC, 🐷)

Herbal Essences Long Term Relationship (LCC, 🐷)

Herbal Essences Totally Twisted Curls and Waves Shampoo with French Lavender Twist & Jade Extracts (LCC, 🐷)

Matrix Biolage Hydrathérapie Hydrating Shampoo (LCC)

Matrix Total Results Curl Boucles (LCC)

Mizani True Textures Cleansing Cream (CC, NS)

Mizani True Textures Curl Balance Moisturizing Sulfate-Free Shampoo (CC, NS)

Motions Moisturizing Cleanser (CC, NS)

Optimum Oil Therapy Ultimate Recovery Shampoo (LCC, 🐷)

Organic Root Stimulator Olive Oil Creamy Aloe Shampoo (CC, 🐷)

Organix Tea Tree Mint Shampoo (CC, NS, 🐷)

Pantene Pro-V Hydrating Curls Shampoo (LCC, 🐷)

Pantene Pro-V Relaxed and Natural Shampoo (LCC, 🐷)

Paul Mitchell Awapuhi Wild Ginger Moisturizing Lather Shampoo (LCC)

Redken Fresh Curls Shampoo (LCC)

SheaMoisture Coconut & Hibiscus Shampoo (CC, NS)

SheaMoisture Organic Raw Shea Butter Moisture Retention Shampoo (CC, NS)

SheaMoisture Yucca & Baobab Thickening Shampoo (CC, NS)

Suave Daily Clarifying Shampoo (LCC, 🐷)

Suave Professionals Rosemary and Mint Shampoo (LCC, 🐷)

Tigi Bed Head Foxy Curls Shampoo (LCC)

Tigi Bed Head Styleshots Hi-Def Curls Shampoo (CC, NS)

Tigi Catwalk Curlesque Defining Shampoo (CC, NS)

Trader Joe's Tea Tree Tingle (CC, 🐷)

Tresemme Vitamin E Moisture Rich (LCC, 🐷)

ONLINE

AG Hair Cosmetics Re: Coil Curl Activating Shampoo (CC, NS)

Aubrey Blue Hydrating Shampoo (CC, NS)

Aubrey Organics GPB Glycogen Protein Balancing Shampoo (CC, NS)

Aubrey Organics Green Tea Clarifying Shampoo (CC, NS)

Aubrey Organics Honeysuckle Rose Moisturizing Shampoo (CC, NS)

Aubrey Organics Rosa Mosqueta Nourishing Shampoo (CC, NS)

Aveda Brilliant Shampoo (CC, NS)

Babo Botanicals Berry Primrose Smooth Detangling Shampoo (CC, NS)

Batia & Aleeza Bio-Natural Shampoo (CC, NS)

BioSilk Silk Therapy Shampoo (CC, NS)

Blended Beauty Soy Cream Shampoo (CC, NS)

Bumble and Bumble Curl Conscious Smoothing Shampoo (CC, NS)

Curly Hair Solutions Silk Shampoo (CC, NS)

Curly Hair Solutions Treatment Shampoo (CC, NS)

DermOrganic Sulfate-Free Conditioning Shampoo with Argan Oil (CC, NS)

DevaCurl or DevaCare Low-Poo (CC, NS)

DevaCurl or DevaCare No-Poo (CC, NS)

shampooing vs. co-washing

To shampoo or to co-wash? That is the question. When we shampoo, we cleanse and usually expect squeaky-clean hair. This is awesome, but it can leave us with a canvas that needs to be remoisturized, deep-treated, detangled, and styled to perfection!

Co-washing often serves as an abbreviated version of your typical shampooing regimen. Co-washing generally consists of using conditioner in place of shampoo. After you rinse out the conditioner, add a leave-in conditioner and/or hairstyling products as you see fit, and voilà! You've co-washed! It's

Elucence Moisture Benefits Shampoo (CC, 🐷, NS, ♡)

Hair Rules Aloe Grapefruit Purifying Shampoo (CC, NS)

Hair Rules Daily Cleansing Cream Moisturizing No Suds Shampoo (CC, NS)

Jane Carter Solution Hydrating Invigorating Shampoo (CC, NS)

KeraCare Natural Textures Cleansing Cream (CC, NS)

Kinky-Curly Come Clean Moisturizing Shampoo (CC, NS)

KMS California Hair Stay Clarify Shampoo (CC, NS)

L'Oréal EverSleek Intense Smoothing Shampoo (CC, NS)

Mahogany Roots Healthy Hair Shampoo Bar (CC, NS)

Matrix Curl Life Shampoo (CC, NS)

Miss Jessie's Super Slip Sudsy Shampoo (CC, NS)

MOP C-System Hydrating Shampoo (CC, NS)

MopTop Gentle Shampoo (CC, NS)

Ojon Ultra Hydrating Shampoo (CC, NS)

Original Moxie Get Clean No-Foam Shampoo (CC, NS)

Ouidad Clear & Gentle Essential Daily Shampoo (CC, NS)

Oyin Grand Poo Bar Succulent Solid Shampoo (CC, NS)

Oyin Honey Wash (CC, NS)

Redken All Soft Shampoo (LCC)

Redken Smooth Down Shampoo (LCC)

Renpure Organics My Pretty Hair Is Parched! Moisturizing Shampoo (CC, NS)

SheaMoisture Organic African Black Soap Deep Cleansing Shampoo (CC, NS)

Terressentials Mud Wash (CC, NS)

Water Bearer Hair Care Super Saturate Shampoo (CC, NS)

Co-washes

As I Am Coconut CoWash Cleansing Conditioner (CC, NS, ♡)

Generic Value Products Detangler (comparable to Paul Mitchell The Conditioner; CC)

Trader Joe's Nourish Spa (CC, 🐷)

Trader Joe's Tea Tree Tingle (CC, 🐷)

Tresemme Naturals Moisture Conditioner (CC, 🐷, ♡)

Yes to Carrots Conditioner (LCC, 🐷)

Yes to Cucumbers Conditioner (LCC, 🐷)

ONLINE

As I Am Cleansing Pudding (CC, NS)

As I Am Coconut CoWash Cleansing Conditioner (CC, NS, ♡)

Avlon KeraCare Natural Textures Cleansing Cream (CC, NS)

Blended Beauty Curl Cleansing Conditioner (CC, NS)

diCesare Oat Cream Moisturizing Hair Wash (CC, NS)

Hamadi Ginger Soymilk Hair Wash (CC, NS)

Mizani True Textures Cleansing Cream Conditioning Curl Wash (CC, NS)

Ouidad Curl Co-wash (CC, NS)

Wen by Chaz Dean Fig Cleansing Conditioner (CC, NS)

Wen by Chaz Dean Sweet Almond Mint Cleansing Conditioner (CC, NS)

that simple and that quick. Co-washes work best for curlies who can't go longer than a few days to a week without washing their hair.

How often do you wash your hair? What do you hope to achieve after you wash it? How does your hair respond to washes? Answer these questions to figure out whether a co-wash and/ or shampoo regimen is best for you. And don't forget to listen to your hair. Don't co-wash if it's practically begging you to shampoo.

CONDITIONERS

Instant Conditioners

Instant conditioner is typically used right after you rinse out your shampoo. Think of it as the second half of your typical shampoo-conditioner combo. Your instant conditioner is supposed to "instantly" moisturize the hair and make it easier to manage. A lot of us in the natural hair community value "slip" when it comes to our conditioners. A good or great conditioner provides easier manipulation when you're trying to comb through your curls. This is referred to as good slip. Some naturals add essential oils to their instant conditioner to give them a little extra slip and added moisture. Instant conditioners are usually rinsed out after a good comb through but can sometimes be used as leave-ins as well.

BRICK AND MORTAR FINDS

Alberto VO5 Moisture Milks Strawberries and Cream Moisturizing Conditioner (LCC, 🐷)

American Cream Conditioner by Lush (CC)

Aussie Moist Conditioner (LCC, 🐷, ♡)

Curls Coconut Sublime Moisturizing Conditioner (CC, 🐷)

Garnier Fructis Triple Nutrition Conditioner (LCC, 🐷)

Giovanni 50:50 Balanced Conditioner (CC, 🐷)

Herbal Essences Hello Hydration Conditioner (LCC, 🐷)

Herbal Essences Long Term Relationship Conditioner (LCC, 🐷)

Herbal Essences Totally Twisted Curls and Waves Conditioner (LCC, 🐷)

Mizani Supreme Oil Conditioner (CC, ♡)

Motions Smoothing Conditioner (CC)

Nexxus Humectress Ultimate Moisturizing Conditioner (LCC)

Pantene Relaxed & Natural Intensive Moisturizing Conditioner (LCC, 🐷)

Paul Mitchell The Detangler (CC)

SheaMoisture Organic Raw Shea Butter Restorative Conditioner (CC, 🐷)

Suave Tropical Coconut Conditioner (LCC, 🐷)

Tigi Bed Head Moisture Maniac Conditioner (CC)

Tigi Bed Head Style Shots Hi-Def Curl Conditioner (LCC)

Tresemme Naturals Moisture Conditioner (CC, 🐷)

Yes to Carrots Conditioner (LCC, 🐷)

Yes to Cucumber Conditioner (LCC, 🐷)

ONLINE

Aubrey GPB Glycogen Protein Balancing Conditioner (CC, 🐷, ♡)

Aveda Be Curly Conditioner (CC)

Blended Beauty Curl Quenching Conditioner (CC)

Curl Junkie Curl Assurance Smoothing Conditioner (CC)

Darcy's Botanicals Pumpkin Seed Moisturizing Conditioner (CC)

DevaCare or DevaCurl One Condition (LCC)

Elucence Moisture Balancing Conditioner (CC, 🐷)

Matrix Curl Life Conditioner (LCC)

Miss Jessie's Crème de la Crème Conditioner (LCC)

MopTop Deep Conditioner (CC)

Ojon Ultra Hydrating Conditioner (LCC)

Ouidad Balancing Rinse (CC)

Oyin Honey Hemp Conditioner (CC)

Spiral Solutions Deeply Decadent Moisturizing Treatment (CC)

Deep Conditioners

Deep conditioners are fantastic for those times when you really need to give your hair some TLC. Regular deep conditioning treatments can yield many positive results, such as moisturizing the hair, thus making it more manageable and restoring much-needed nutrients, such as protein, to the strands. Deep conditioners are usually left on the hair anywhere from three minutes to forty-five minutes. Be sure to read and follow the directions given on each product, as no two conditioners work exactly alike. Nikki recommends deep conditioning at every wash session for the most benefits.

BRICK AND MORTAR FINDS

Aphogee Keratin 2 Minute Reconstructor (LCC, 🐷)

Aussie 3 Minute Miracle Deeeeep Conditioner (LCC, 🐷)

Aussie 3 Minute Miracle Reconstructor for Damaged Hair (LCC, 🐷)

Carol's Daughter Black Vanilla Hair Smoothie (CC)

Carol's Daughter Olive Oil Infusion Softening and Detangling At-Home Hair Treatment (CC)

Carol's Daughter Tui Hair Smoothie (CC)

Curls Curl Ecstasy Hair Tea Conditioner (CC)

Garnier Fructis Sleek & Shine Fortifying Deep Conditioner 3 Minute Masque (LCC, 🐷)

L'Oréal EverSleek Smoothing Deep Conditioner (LCC, 🐷)

Lustrasilk Shea Butter Cholesterol (LCC, 🐷)

Matrix Biolage Conditioning Balm (CC)

Motions Deep Conditioning Mask (CC)

Organic Root Stimulator Olive Oil Replenishing Conditioner (LCC, 🐷)

Pantene Curly Hair Series Deep Moisturizing Treatment (LCC, 🐷)

Paul Mitchell Super-Charged
Conditioner (LCC)

SheaMoisture Organic Raw

Shea Butter Deep Treatment
Masque (CC, 🐷)

AG Hair Cosmetics Conditioner
Deep Reconstructing
Treatment (LCC)

Aubrey Organics Honeysuckle
Rose Moisturizing Conditioner
(CC)

Aubrey Organics White
Camellia (CC)

Bee Mine Bee-U-Ti-Ful Deep
Conditioner (CC)

Curl Junkie Hibiscus and
Banana (CC)

Curl Junkie Rehab
Moisturizing Hair Treatment
(CC)

Darcy's Botanicals Pumpkin
Seed Moisturizing Conditioner
(CC)

DevaCurl Heaven in Hair
Intense Moisture Treatment
(CC)

Jessicurl Deep Conditioner
(CC)

Jessicurl Too Shea! Extra
Moisturizing Conditioner
(CC)

Miss Jessie's Rapid Recovery
Treatment (LCC)

Mixed Chicks Deep Conditioner
(LCC)

MopTop Deep Conditioner
(CC)

MyHoneyChild Olive You
(CC, ♡)

Ouidad 12 Minute Deep
Treatment (CC)

Organic Root Stimulator Hair
Mayonnaise (CC, 🐷)

Wen by Chaz Dean Fig Oil (CC)

Leave-in Conditioners

Leave-in conditioners are for regular hair maintenance. They
can be used every day or as needed. A good leave-in conditioner

will provide your hair with the moisture and nourishment it needs until your next wash, condition, or deep conditioning treatment.

BRICK AND MORTAR FINDS

Cantu Shea Butter Leave-in Conditioner Repair Cream (LCC, 🐷)

Carol's Daughter Black Vanilla Leave-In Conditioner (CC)

Carol's Daughter Hair Milk (CC)

Curls Quenched Curls Moisturizer (CC)

Garnier Fructis Sleek & Shine Leave-In Conditioning Cream (LCC, 🐷)

Giovanni Direct Leave-In Conditioner (CC, 🐷)

Giovanni Smooth as Silk Conditioner (CC, 🐷)

Infusium 23 Leave In Conditioner (LCC, 🐷)

Kinky-Curly Knot Today (CC)

L'Oréal EverSleek Humidity Defying Leave-In Crème (LCC, 🐷)

Paul Mitchell The Cream (LCC)

Redken Extreme Anti-Snap Leave-in Treatment (LCC)

SheaMoisture Organic Coconut Hibiscus Curl and Style Milk (CC, 🐷)

Tigi Bed Head Ego Boost Leave-In Conditioner (LCC)

Tigi Catwalk Curlesque Leave-In Conditioner (LCC)

Yes to Carrots Leave-In Conditioner (LCC, 🐷)

ONLINE

AG Hair Cosmetics Fast Food Leave On Conditioner (CC)

BioSilk Silk Therapy (LCC)

Bumble and Bumble Leave-In Conditioner (LCC)

Curl Junkie Curl Assurance Smoothing Lotion (CC, ♡)

Curly Hair Solutions Silk Leave-In Conditioner (CC)

Darcy's Botanicals Daily Leave-In Conditioner (CC)

Darcy's Botanicals Herbal Leave-In Conditioning Spritz (CC)

Darcy's Botanicals Organic Coconut & Aloe Moisture Pudding (CC)

Davines De-Stress Shelter Leave-in (LCC, ♡)

Elucence Moisture Balancing Conditioner (CC, 🐷)

Karen's Body Beautiful Sweet Ambrosia Leave-In Conditioner (CC)

Karen's Body Beautiful Hair Nectar (CC)

Mixed Chicks Leave-in Conditioner (LCC)

Oyin Hair Dew (CC)

Oyin Juices and Berries Nourishing Herbal Leave-In (CC)

Salerm 21 (LCC)

Star Lacio Lacio High Shine Leave-in Conditioner (LCC, 🐷)

OILS AND SEALANTS

Sealing the hair (especially the ends) is a very important practice in any hair care regimen. In order for sealing to be effective, use a water-based moisturizer (a conditioner or a cream that has water as its first ingredient) and then seal with a butter or an oil. The molecules in most butters or oils are too large to pass into the hair, so they stick to the outside of the shaft, trapping in the rich goodness of the moisturizer. Reversing those two steps will lead to dry hair. Sealing not only keeps your hair looking fabulous but will also keep your ends protected.

BRICK AND MORTAR FINDS

Argan oil (CC)

Carol's Daughter Hair Balm (CC)

Carol's Daughter Khoret Amen Hair Oil (CC)

Carol's Daughter Lisa's Hair Elixir (CC)

Carol's Daughter Mimosa Hair Honey (CC)

Carol's Daughter Olive Oil Infusion Softening and Detangling At-Home Hair Treatment (CC)

CHI Organics Oil Spray Oil Treatment for Hair and Skin (LCC)

Curls Champagne & Caviar Curl Elixir (CC)

Jamaican Black Castor Oil (CC, 🐷)

Jane Carter Nourish and Shine (CC)

Redken UV Rescue Protective Oil (LCC)

SheaMoisture Organic Raw Shea Butter Reconstructive Elixir (CC)

Unrefined shea butter (CC, 🐷)

Vatika oil (LCC)

Wild Growth Hair Oil (LCC)

ONLINE

AfroVeda Emu Oil (CC)

AfroVeda Hibiscus Hair Infusion Herbal Oil (CC)

AfroVeda Priti Bodhi Rice Bran Herbal Hair Oil (CC)

AfroVeda SunSilk Citrus Herbal Hair Oil (CC)

AG Hair Cosmetics The Oil (CC)

Avlon KeraCare Essential Oils (LCC)

Avlon KeraCare Oil Sheen (LCC)

Bee Mine Hair Growth Serum Strawberry Kiwi (CC)

Blended Beauty Natural Hair Oil (CC)

Cantu Shea Butter No Drip Hair and Scalp Oil (LCC, 🐷)

Carol's Daughter Healthy Hair Butter (CC)

Carol's Daughter Tui Hair Oil (CC)

Couture Colour Pequi Oil Treatment (LCC)

Curls of the World Gypsy Magic Hair Growth Oil (LCC)

Cush Cosmetics 97% Organic Argan Oil (CC)

Darcy's Botanicals Cherry Kernel Nectar Hair & Body Oil (CC, 🐷)

Darcy's Botanicals Cocoa Bean Natural Hair & Body Oil (CC, 🐷)

Darcy's Botanicals Juicy Peach Kernel Nectar (CC, 🐷)

Darcy's Botanicals Organic Coconut & Hibiscus Conditioning Oil (CC, 🐷)

Darcy's Botanicals Sweet Apricot Kernel Hair & Body Oil (CC, 🐷)

Davines Absolute Beautifying Potion (LCC)

De Fabulous Acai Oil Treatment (LCC)

DermOrganic Intensive Hair Repair Masque with Argan Oil (CC)

Eden Body Works All Natural Peppermint and Tea Tree Hair Oil (CC)

Finickey Glossing Serum Natural Hair Oil (CC)

HairVeda Vatika Frosting (CC)

HPO Spa Treatments Happy Scalp (CC)

Jane Carter Solution Scalp Nourishing Serum Scalp Fortifier (CC)

Jessicurl Oil Blend for Softer Hair (CC)

Jessicurl Stimulating Scalp Massage Oil (CC)

John Frieda Frizz-Ease Rebuild Restructuring Micro-Oil Therapy (LCC)

Jojoba oil (CC, 🐷)

Karen's Body Beautiful Butter Love (CC)

Karen's Body Beautiful Heavenly Jojoba Hair Oil (CC)

Marc Anthony Strictly Curls Oil of Morocco (LCC)

Mira Herbals Hair Oil (CC)

Mizani Confiderm Scalp Oil (LCC)

Mizani Supreme Oil (CC)

Moroccanoil Treatment (LCC)

MyHoneyChild Intensive Oil Treatment (CC)

MyHoneyChild Old Fashioned Hair Grease (CC)

NU-GRO All-Natural Liquid Hair Gro Oil (CC)

Organix Renewing Moroccan Argan Oil Penetrating Oil (LCC)

Original Moxie Hair Bling (CC)

Ouidad Mongongo Oil (CC, ♡)

Oyin Handmade Burnt Sugar Pomade (CC)

Oyin Handmade Sugar Berry Pomade (CC, ♡)

Oyin Handmade Whipped Shea (CC, 🐷)

PhytoSpecific Revitalizing Oil (CC)

Qhemet Amla Oil Nourishing Pomade (CC)

Qhemet Biologics Amla Oil Nourishing Pomade (CC)

Qhemet Biologics Castor & Moringa Softening Serum (CC)

Qhemet Biologics Olive & Honey Hydrating Balm (CC)

Redken Real Control Mineral Elixir Dazzling Smoothing Oil (LCC)

Shea Terra Organics Baobab Face and Body Oil (CC)

Shea Terra Organics Certified Organic Tamanu Oil (CC)

Sofn'free GroHealthy Milk Protein and Olive Oil Three-Layer Growth Oil (LCC)

Sunny Isle Jamaican Black Castor Oil (CC)

Wen by Chaz Dean Cucumber Aloe Oil (CC)

Wen by Chaz Dean Fig Oil (CC)

Wen by Chaz Dean Sweet Almond Mint Oil (CC)

Zuri Natural Moisture-Rising Hair Oil (CC)

OUR FAVORITE "KITCHEN" OILS

Virgin coconut oil (CC, 🐷)

Extra virgin olive oil (CC, 🐷)

Grape seed oil (CC, 🐷)

STYLERS

Using a styler is a less essential step in a natural hair care routine—gels, curl creams, and mousses fall in this category. The use of a styler often results in a more controlled, sleeker, less voluminous look. If you like big, fluffy hair, you may want to skip this step and opt for a light-hold styling product or find a conditioner that has a little hold. Many of the products listed below are lighter stylers. Nikki loves big hair.

BRICK AND MORTAR FINDS

Aloe vera gel (CC, 🐷)

Aubrey Organics Mandarin Magic Ginkgo Leaf and Ginseng Root Hair Jelly (CC)

Aveda Light Elements Defining Whip (CC)

Biolage Gelée (CC)

Eco Styler Gel (LCC, 🐷)

Garnier Fructis Cream Gel (LCC, 🐷)

Garnier Fructis Sleek & Shine Leave-In Conditioning Cream (LCC, 🐷)

Herbal Essences Totally Twisted Curl Boosting Mousse (LCC, 🐷)

Herbal Essences Totally Twisted Curl Scrunching Gel (LCC, 🐷)

Jamaican Mango & Lime Locking Gel (LCC, 🐷)

Jane Carter Wrap and Roll (CC)

Kinky-Curly Curling Custard (CC)

L.A. Looks Curl Looks Gel (LCC, 🐷)

L.A. Looks Sport Look Gel (dark blue; LCC, 🐷)

Motions Hydrate My Curls Pudding (CC)

Organic Root Stimulator Lock & Twist Gel (LCC, 🐷)

Pantene Curl Defining Scrunching Mousse (LCC, 🐷)

Samy Big Curls Curl Defining Cream (LCC, 🐷)

Samy Get Curls Re-Energizing Potion (LCC, 🐷)

Shea Moisture Coconut and Hibiscus Curl Enhancing Smoothie (CC, 🐷)

Tigi Catwalk Curlesque Curls Rock Amplifier (LCC)

ONLINE

Afroveda PUR Whipped Hair Jelly (CC)

Alagio Crazy Curl Curl Enhancer Balm (CC)

As I Am Curling Jelly Coil and Curl Definer (CC)

As I Am Twist Defining Cream (CC)

Aussie Sydney Smooth Tizz No Frizz Gel (LCC, 🐷)

Aveda Be Curly Curl Enhancer Lotion (CC)

Aveda Brilliant Humectant Pomade (LCC)

Batia & Aleeza Bio-Herbal Mineral Sculpting Gel (CC)

Bee Mine Bee Hold Curly Butter (CC)

Beyond the Zone Noodle Head Curling Creme (LCC)

Blended Beauty Curly Frizz Pudding (CC)

Blended Beauty Happy Nappy (CC)

Curl Junkie Coffee-Coco Curl Creme Lite (CC)

Curl Junkie Curl Assurance Aloe Fix Hair Styling Gel (CC)

Curl Junkie Curl Assurance Smoothing Gellie (CC)

Curl Junkie Curl Queen Gel (CC)

Curl Junkie Curls in a Bottle (CC)

Curlisto Control Gel II (CC)

Curlisto Structura Lotion (CC)

Curls Curl Gel-les'c (CC)

Curls Curl Souffle (CC)

Curls Quenched Curls Moisturizer (CC)

Curls Souffle (CC)

Curls Whipped Cream (CC)

DevaCurl MirrorCurls (LCC)

DevaCurl Mist-er Right (CC)

DevaCurl Set It Free (LCC)

Frédéric Fekkai Luscious Curls Curl Enhancing Lotion (LCC, CC)

Fruit of the Earth Aloe Gel (CC, 🐷)

Giovanni L.A. Natural Styling Gel (CC, 🐷)

Hair Rules Hydrating Finishing Cream (LCC)

Innersense Quiet Calm Curl Control (CC)

Jane Carter Solution Condition & Sculpt (CC)

Jessicurl Confident Coils Styling Solution (CC)

Jessicurl Gelebration Spray (CC)

Jessicurl Rockin' Ringlets (CC)

John Frieda Frizz-Ease Curl Dreams Curl Perfecting Spray (LCC)

Kinky-Curly Spiral Spritz Natural Styling Serum (CC)

Kiss My Face Upper Management Gel (CC)

LaBella Lots of Curls Gel (LCC, 🐷)

L'Oréal Studio Springing Curls Mousse (CC)

Marc Anthony Strictly Curls Curl Defining Lotion (CC)

Matrix Curl Life Contouring Milk (LCC)

Miss Jessie's Baby Buttercreme (LCC)

Miss Jessie's Curly Buttercreme (LCC)

Miss Jessie's Curly Meringue (LCC)

Miss Jessie's Stretch Silkening Cream (LCC)

MOP Glisten High Shine Pomade (CC)

Original Moxie Luxe Locks Styling and Shine (CC)

Ouidad Climate Control Heat & Humidity Gel (CC)

Ouidad Curl Quencher Hydrafusion Curl Cream (CC, ♡)

Ouidad Curl Quencher Moisturizing Gel (CC)

Oyin Shine and Define Styling Serum (CC)

Oyin Whipped Pudding (CC)

Pantene Pro-V Curl Defining Scrunching Gel (LCC, 🐷)

Paul Mitchell Express Style Round Trip (LCC)

Qhemet Biologics Honeybush Hair Tea Soft Hold Gel (CC)

Qhemet Biologics Olive & Honey Hydrating Balm (CC)

Redken Fresh Curls Curl Refiner (LCC)

Spiral Solutions Curl Enhancing Jelly (CC, LCC)

Spiral Solutions Firm Holding Styling Gel (LCC, CC)

Tigi Bed Head Control Freak Frizz Control and Straightener Serum (LCC)

Tigi Bed Head Candy Fixations Totally Baked Volumizing and Prepping Hair Meringue (CC, ♡)

PHOTO CREDITS

Grateful acknowledgment is made for use of the following photos:

Page ix: Daniel Reichert; page xiv: Dr. Eugene Walton Jr.; page 9: Charnele A. Hylton; page 13 (*top to bottom*): Antoinette Henry, Angelica Moss; page 14: Monique Herbert (*Naturally Monique*); page 18: Marie Smith; page 22: Chatel Theagene; page 28: Monique King-Viehland; page 31 (*top to bottom*): Autumn, Gaye Glasspie; page 34: Ebony Joy Wilkins; page 39: Jalisa Roberts; page 40: Onyeka Ifejika; page 43: Ni-Kiya Alleyne; page 46: *Natural-ness: A Journey Through the Lengths*; pages 55–56, 62: Jessica Lewis; pages 58, 86–87: Alexandra Smith (*The Good Hair Blog*); page 64: Reanell Frederick; page 65 (*top to bottom*): Nikevia Bowie, Briaan Barron; page 69: Gaye Glasspie; page 76: Sherrell Dorsey; page 77: www.TheWriteCurlDiary.com; pages 88–91: Savvy Brown; page 91 (*bottom*): Shan'Terika Remo; page 92 (*top to bottom*): Fern Illidge, Chantel Nattiel; page 94: Ebony Clark; page 99: Shelli A. Gillis; page 118: Dr. Eugene Walton Jr.; page 123: TiaShauntee; page 124: Dr. Eugene Walton Jr.; page 127: Chime Edwards (*Hair Crush*); page 129: Charnika Jett; page 132: Dr. Eugene Walton Jr.; page 133 (*top to bottom*): Dr. Eugene Walton Jr., Shelli A. Gillis; page 134: Danielle Faust; page 136 (*top to bottom*): Erica James, Desiree Brandon, Brandi Preston; page 138: Asia Lynn; page 142: Nadine Afia (*Girls Love Your Curls*); pages 153–154: *Wise Curls* (Angela Pierre); page 158: Tim Dallesandro; page 163: Christian Hibbard; page 168: Jamyla Bennu; page 171: Dr. Eugene Walton Jr.; page 172: Amber Wright; page 173 (*top to bottom*): Michelle Parker, Lesa H. Elder; page 174 (*top to bottom*): Tenesha Bailey, Ylandus Roundy; page 176: Dr. Eugene Walton Jr.; page 179: Shanti Mayers; page 183: Topshelf Junior.